The Bread Crumb Trail: A Journey Through Chronic Illness to Wholeness

Dedication

To *my* Grandpa—thank you for the journey, for the lessons.
To the many friends who have walked beside me, your support has been a constant light along my path. Each of you have been instrumental in your own way! 🤚 Thank you for guiding me to a whole new version of myself and for always believing in me, even when I didn't. (Deb, Lauren, Tami, Danny—thank you for your unwavering friendship and encouragement.)
And to Tank—who made me use those stinky essential oils so many years ago! You were right, and now I can't imagine my healing journey without them. To my family - Thank you for giving me space and support to pursue these unconventional approaches.

Much love

Table Of Contents:

Introduction

THE "IMPACT"

From as early as I can remember I have always felt things deeply. I perceive people and animals (and sometimes objects) in scenes and metaphor. This is how I thought everyone perceived each other. So, in my mind, there was no need to ask questions because that was just normal for everyone, right? It wasn't until I got to be a little older and in grade school that I found out that was not so. I feel others' as if they radiate energy. I perceive them as a gentle breeze, a dark cloud, a color, object or a place (such as a sunny field). The more I interact with someone, the stronger "their feeling" becomes to me. Family and close friends have a feeling that is specific to them....much like wearing a signature perfume or cologne. My interpretation of their feelings changes depending on how they are being influenced by their environment. These sensations change based on their mood, environment and circumstances. Meaning, if someone usually feels light and sunny to me and I run into them and they are dealing with something that is upsetting them, I may perceive them as a dark cloud, or a heavy sensation which usually catches my attention. Then I may pick up on the specific feelings.... (conflict, anxiety, hurt, embarrassment, etc) This sensitivity is sometimes called being an 'empath,' a person who deeply feels and interprets others' emotions.

I started grade school in 1980. This was before the days of social media, cell phones, etc. If your friends weren't in your class with you, you didn't know if they were absent from school until lunch or recess. I recall being in the 4th grade and sitting at the lunch table with my friends. We were debating if one of our group members was held up in class and just hadn't arrived at the lunch table or if she was absent for the day. I recall closing my eyes and searching for her "*feeling*". (Not realizing at the time, I was searching for her energetically.) When I opened my eyes, I casually commented, *"I don't feel her, she's not here."* To my surprise, my comments prompted a large amount of ridicule from my friends. "What do you mean *"you don't feel her"*?, they asked. And I naively repeated *"I don't feel her, do you?"* There's no need to carry on the remainder of the story. The bottom line was my friends made fun of me, calling me weird, creepy, bad, strange, and many other adjectives. The lesson I learned that day was to never discuss how I "felt people". I also began working diligently to suppress the way I perceived others. Thinking somehow it was bad..... That I was bad. This unique "sensitivity" shaped how I navigated all relationships, often causing both connection issues and confusion.

By feeling things deeply, I could often feel the intent or emotion behind other's words or actions. From birth, the people I could feel the strongest, were my mom and dad, my 2 brothers, my Aunt and Uncle (Pat and Bud) and my Grandfather (on my mother's side who I affectionately called "Grandpa.") They were my safety, security and my "inner circle". These were the BEDROCK on which I had begun to build the foundation of my life. They were my 'constants'. They would ALWAYS be there.

I could clearly feel the love from my family, and in some cases, the lack of love from other members. Where many children need to be hugged and cuddled to feel love and affection, it was just *known* for me, a common knowledge. I never doubted it. Because of this, I was not overly affectionate, nor did I like to be touched often. Touching others can intensify what I pick up off of them. Sometimes it is very LOUD and overwhelming energetically. Again, as a child I assumed everyone felt life like this.

My grandfather was the only person I could touch and feel like everything was muffled. He softened the LOUD that was always around me. In my mind he was a warm pulsating blue orb. Like a heartbeat. He had a strong feeling that was comforting and compassionate. Much like a warm blanket out of the dryer. Very loving and very kind. He always referred to me as "*my Angel*" and his words only proved to emphasize the FEELINGS I perceived from him.

My Grandpa was a little guy. Barely over 5 feet tall. But, to me he was the BIGGEST person in the room. His energy was very dominant and filled a large space. By the time I was 7 yrs old I was almost as big as him so I found the arm of his chair to be the best place for me to sit so I could be near him. In almost all of my childhood pictures with my Grandpa, I am either standing beside him or perched on the arm of his chair.

Unfortunately, being so young, I had little life experience to pull from. I could FEEL people, but I was naively unaware of the "dark side" of life. *Illness, death, loss.* I assumed everyone felt each other in this manner so I never thought to ask questions. Life was perfect. I loved those closest to me and I could FEEL their love for me. Unfortunately, this created a false sense of security. *I assumed this was how it would ALWAYS be.*

I was unaware that my grandfather was ill. As it was, he had been diagnosed with cancer when I was 4 or 5 years old. He had been told he had *6 months to live.* He was a determined man and proceeded to live for another 6 years. During this time, his health continually declined resulting in his being placed in a nursing home the last year of his life. I recall being so angry that no one in my family loved him enough to take care of him. THIS WAS NOT THE CASE! But as a child, this was MY PERCEPTION of events. We would go to the nursing home every weekend to see him and I recall thinking as we walked through the halls of that sad, smelly place that "all those people are here because no one loves them or wants to take care of them." I remember standing in the hallway outside my grandpa's room one afternoon. I was so angry we were leaving him there yet again. I made a promise to myself that day! As soon as I was 18 I was going to come get my Grandpa and take him to live with me. I would take care of him. I would take care of ALL of my family. No one I loved would ever have to go to a nursing home ever again.

Such a serious SELF PROMISE to be made at 8 and ½ yrs old.

Before my grandfather passed, his presence was my comfort. He often told me, 'You are my Angel,' I felt secure, but I was unaware of the weight of those words at the time. I was 9, when he passed. I had NO IDEA how these events would set the stage for chronic illness later in life.

****

October 1982, I knew something was very wrong. I could feel the weight of "something bad" in the air but I had no idea, explanation, or context to go on. I just "felt it". I could feel that my mom was stressed and upset, but no understanding why.

Side note: It is a very confusing thing for a child to FEEL things but not have words or ideas to explain them. To HEAR the words someone was speaking but not FEEL the same intention off of them. Sometimes I would feel quite the opposite.

To hear "Nothing is wrong "but to FEEL the atmosphere of the room and just KNOW that I was being lied to. Lies are bad, right? Why would my family LIE to me? It took years to learn they weren't LYING..... Not intentionally. They were

Back to October - We were going to my grandma's apartment. I knew it wasn't our normal time to go visit grandpa. I was also mad because my mom made me stay with my dad and brothers while she went to the nursing home. I never missed an opportunity to see my grandpa, so the fact someone was going without me was "UNFAIR" in my mind.

I can clearly recall sitting on the couch watching cartoons and something felt very wrong. I couldn't tell WHAT, it was something I had never felt.....or NOT FELT before.

Very shortly after I had felt this "shift", is when the news came that my grandpa had died. It was life altering for me. I had never experienced "death" yet. I had NO COMPREHENSION of what death was. The finality. The magnitude. The IMPACT it would have on my life. The fact that it was the passing of one of the most important people in my life caused the solid foundation of my existence to be shaken. To crumble. People died? They LEFT YOU? No "good bye"? No explanation? I wont say I had never had a panic attack prior to this event. (I was a very anxious child.) But I can say I don't recall it. What I do recall, is that I began having them quite frequently after my grandpa passed. Almost daily.

It is important to point out here that this ONE EVENT is not what caused all of my illness or maladaptive coping mechanisms. It was a large portion, but not the whole. No ONE EVENT is the "whole".

The point of this is to convey how my diving into my OWN STORY has provided me with certain points and events that were contributory to my illness. There were many other contributing factors that worked to support my disease path and others that I created from my skewed perceptions. -More on that later.

One of the strongest FEELINGS I had known in my life was no longer there. I felt unstable. Lost. Off balance. Unsafe. Empty. Hollow. ANGRY! Very, very angry. An all-consuming anger that permeated every cell of my body. The minute I was given the news, I went into a blind rage. It truly felt "out of body". I completely destroyed my grandmother's kitchen. I pulled out drawers, threw things, opened every drawer and threw the contents. I screamed. I cried. I collapsed. I went numb.

I was in a fog. A numbing, all consuming mental fog.

I don't recall the timeline of events. I only remember being at the Funeral home and seeing my grandpa in "the box" as I called it. I could SEE him. But I couldn't FEEL him anymore. It was so confusing and scary. It was beyond anything I knew at the time. The pain was so overwhelming and devastating. I determined right then and there I would NEVER feel this again!

I clearly recall standing in the funeral home pushing the air away from me with my hands and telling myself that *"if I didn't love people, it wouldn't hurt me if this happened to anyone else."* I pushed everything away. Nothing was allowed close. That DAY I put things in motion that would begin the destruction of my body. I had made the CONSCIOUS DECISION to "not feel things". I stuffed everything down deep inside and ignored it.

I refused to cry anymore about it. I REFUSED to grieve. I refused to "let it go". I took the anger and held on to it as if it were my identity..... And so, it became my identity.

A "Sensitive" – 1. A person with the ability to understand the experiences or feelings of others outside your own perspective. 2. One who can comprehend the mental or emotional state of another.

This was a word I had never heard until I was in my 40's. I had no comprehension of what that meant or how that impacted me. I just knew I could often pick up on how others felt. I knew I could stand in a classroom and FEEL how everyone perceived me. I knew when someone was lying to me. Who was friend, who was foe. Who liked me, who didn't. I could feel who was listening and who wasn't when I had to give a report in class. It is such an intimidating feeling to be in front of your peers and FEEL (to some degree) what they are thinking about you. Adolescents are very critical. This can be very damaging to an empath. Especially one who has never had anyone to help them navigate what they are experiencing. Such was my case.

I have come to understand far more about myself in this way. I have also come to realize I have many spiritual gifts that God had been trying to bring to my awareness for quite some time. I have embraced what I once feared was mental illness.

Being sensitive left me in a vulnerable state for many years. I didn't understand just how DEEPLY I felt things. I didn't understand why I would be heavily impacted by things that seemed to roll off of others. I honestly thought I had some underlying mental illness. I also had no idea that as a sensitive, you need to perfect 'protecting your own energy.' All of these things, along with my maladaptive coping mechanisms and life experiences were contributing factors to the chronic conditions I would come to be labeled with by conventional medicine.

Fast forward to June of 2017. I was 43 years old. I had been struggling with a series of symptoms that were becoming physically limiting for me. Bilateral joint pain in my ankles, hips, shoulders and wrists. I was always short of breath. I was using my inhaler 6-10 times a DAY because I felt like I couldn't take a deep breath. EVER. I was susceptible to any cold or virus of the respiratory tract that came my direction. *I had made an appointment with my PCP and so, here I sat in his office waiting to get the results of my recent testing.*

Being a nurse, I had already drawn my own conclusion and he only proved to confirm my suspicions. I was DIAGNOSED with LUPUS. I was told I was experiencing a rapid decline and at my current rate I would be in a wheelchair and "probably on oxygen" by the time I was 50yrs old. This was terrifying! It was also unacceptable to me!

I had taken a position as a nurse in a Functional Medicine office when I was 40. I had spent the 3 years BEFORE the diagnosis learning about holistic medicine and how, given the right conditions, that the body can heal itself. I refused to go on medication for my symptoms. My PCP was supportive but also felt that it was a bad decision given how much pain I was in and how quickly my condition had deteriorated from the initial manifestation of symptoms.

I wanted to pursue a NATURAL route and work to HEAL my body. Not start medications that would potentially harm my body in other ways and only work to compound my problems. However, I promised him that I would return and START the TREATMENT of his choice if I got no relief from my symptoms. We decided 3 months was a fair amount of time to allow me to "look at alternative options."

I met with the doctor I worked for that afternoon and got a game plan in place. I also began working with our in-house dietitian and completely altered my diet. Within 3 weeks my pain was 50% better. In 3 months my pain was 80% better. I maintained myself at 80%

improvement for quite some time, but deep in my soul I knew there was MORE. It laid beyond food and supplements. I found the 'MORE' in addressing suppressed emotions and traumas through meditation and the use of ESSENTIAL OILS. These gems facilitate healing and restoration at the spiritual and emotional level. In later chapters, I explore how these modalities helped reconnect my mind, body, and spirit.

Needless to say, I never started the medications my PCP had recommended....I started a journey. A journey that has allowed me to begin the healing process. And allowed for something that was unexpected to me...... I began to FIND ME.

This journey has been exciting, scary, empowering, happy, sad, frustrating and intriguing along with hundreds of other emotions along the way. It has been an ongoing adventure in which I have grown and evolved through trial and error. I have come to understand that I am a 'sensitive person', what all that entails, and how it impacts (positively AND negatively) the healing process. I also know that there is no ONE METHOD that heals you completely. We are LAYERED BEINGS, and therefore; we heal "in layers."

Healing is a PROCESS, not an END GOAL to reach. You may have a specific issue that you want to improve, heal or focus on, but once that area is improved there will be another behind it that needs JUST AS MUCH focus and attention. It can be a slow and overwhelming process in the beginning. But, once you understand the way it works, it becomes much easier to navigate.

Suppressed emotions had become my identity, and it took years to unravel their impact. Through this book, I hope to guide others toward their own healing.

XO- Angel

1.

In A Nutshell

Our body is an AMAZING creation! From 2 cells it forms this complex and beautiful physical shell made up of trillions of cells. All of these cells have different functions and programming. There are electrical impulses and currents, it is surrounded by an energy field. It has cells that nourish and oxygenate and cells that fight pathogens and "clean house". Cells that, given the right environment, enable the body to overcome almost ANYTHING that comes at it. (Over 200 different types of cells)

This PHYSICAL body also has a MIND and SPIRIT. When these 3 parts are in unison, the body is cohesive and functions optimally. Unfortunately our society has perfected the "breakdown" of this trinity. Creating responses in our BE-ing that contribute to DIS-ease and chronic illness. Given enough time, these responses lay the groundwork for terrible outcomes. (Autoimmune illness, mental health disorders, organ malfunction, or even cancer. At any given time, our body is combatting mutated cells that could potentially turn into something malevolent. Often, our system prevails, however if the trinity that is the human BE-ing is not brought back into balance, eventually the system may fail in its endeavors. We live in a society that bombards us daily with OVERSTIMULATION. At birth parents are placing cell phones and ipads in cribs... We are only proving to make this overall DISCONNECT and breakdown in the MIND, BODY, and SPIRIT even worse. Let's discuss how this impacts the physical body...

Threat:
1. a statement of an intention to inflict pain, injury, damage, or other hostile action on someone in retribution for something done or not done
2. a person or thing likely to cause damage or danger

PHYSICAL-

When we perceive a physical threat, the body switches into Fight or Flight mode. (Ex: a menacing dog comes in your yard and begins to growl at you and show its teeth- you body immediately determines **DANGER** and prepares to run away or stand and fight. However, when we live in a state of "STRESS", our brain is interpreting things as DANGER that are NOT DANGEROUS. This is because we are actually living in SURVIVAL mode. The body then works to generate a large amount of energy to face whatever THREAT has been perceived. The pupils dilate so we can "see better". The heart and respiratory rate increase so we can run/fight or hide. Glucose is dumped into the bloodstream, so that we have more energy available to our cells. And blood flow is directed to our extremities and away from our internal organs. The immune system surges initially and then is repressed over time as adrenaline and cortisol flood the body. Circulation is rerouted from CREATIVE thought and increases our instinctual responses. All of this happens so that we can INSTANTLY REACT.

Short term this is how we are designed and how we SHOULD respond to an immediate threat. Once we are away from the **danger**. The body should calm and return to a state of calm.

Living in a state of stress is not optimal or sustainable for the body. When we stay in a state of fight or flight, we don't switch back to rest and digest.... The body becomes"STUCK".

Our body is NOT designed to live in "survival mode" long term. This state, over time, becomes physically destructive. With our brain functioning on a more primitive (instinctual) level, it causes us to think and react fast and without all the information at times. The chemicals of stress are what alter our internal state and set the stage for cellular aging, DIS-ease and death.

MIND-

The most difficult language to communicate is our feelings. From birth, we are taught to suppress our feelings. We are told to "stop whining", "stop complaining", "quit crying, be quiet", etc. Because of our "programming", we suppress, repress, ignore and hide the troubling emotions that are either so painful and overwhelming they consume us, or they are so traumatic we bury them thinking they will go away.

Thoughts and feelings are energy. Everything in the Universe is energy. All energy has a measurable vibration. All feelings/emotions have a vibrational frequency. This can be a positive energy (healing energy) or a negative energy (destructive energy).

Our body does NOT understand time in the sense that we do. The body doesn't know the difference in something that happens today versus 30 years ago. Just by THINKING about an event or situation, by replaying it over and over, our BODY becomes STUCK in this energetic loop that keeps replaying, reliving and PHYSICALLY EXPERIENCING this event over and over.

The same emotions and hormones that occurred during the initial event are produced every time we replay the ordeal in our mind. Once, twice, thirty times a day.... Every "replay" causes the same release of emotions/hormones in the body. Over time, the body will develop an ADDICTION to these emotions and chemicals. No matter how awful the event was, the persistent flooding of the body with these emotions can create a dependency on them, just like an addict develops with drugs and alcohol.

This destructive thought process is called RUMINATION.

> *RUMINATION - A repetitive negative thought process that plays continuously in the mind. (reliving an event, replaying an upsetting conversation, etc) **Rumination causes our body to***

We get caught up in these cycles because we feel like we have no choice. We don't even realize what our thoughts are doing to us. So here we are, stuck in a particular mindset, because our brain has become hardwired due to our thought patterns. If we resolve to no longer replay these painful memories and events from our past - we begin to interrupt our harmful subconscious thoughts.

Emotions are the chemical outcome of past events. As we perceive events and situations, clusters of neurons receive this information. It is fed into networks and as it becomes sealed into a pattern, the brain creates a CHEMICAL that is sent through the entire body. This "chemical" is called an emotion.

We don't usually recall events well by memory alone, we recall how we FELT during the event which clarifies and enhances the memory. The stronger the emotion, the stronger the change in our body. When the body perceives a STRONG emotional response to a person or situation, it "takes a recording" of that event, this is a MEMORY. Memories become embedded in our mind and are 'frozen in time' so to speak. The experience of this event becomes imprinted in our cells and the emotion is stored somewhere in the body. This is how past events can become a contributor to our physical BE-ing. We store these emotions (anger, fear, grief, etc) in different areas of the body.

To give you an example of what emotions resonate with what organs:

> *Anger —> Liver*
> *Sadness —> Heart and Lungs*
> *Fear —> Kidneys/Liver/Gallbladder*
> *Grief —> Lungs*
> *Anxiety —> Heart/Lungs*
> *Anxiety/Fear/Anger/Nervousness —> "the Gut"*

As you can see, negative emotions can really impact our bodies.

What we have discussed so far is how emotions are created from events we have encountered. Let's go a step further. Some of our feelings were established BEFORE we were born...When we were in our mothers womb, many emotions SHE experienced created hormones. These hormones may have impacted our BE-ing as well.

In the same manner we received life sustaining nutrients from her, the emotions and chemicals she experienced due to her situation and environment could (and often does) cause us to establish incorrect perceptions. At 24 weeks of gestation the fetus can HEAR. It can perceive tones and voices. Not only is it HEARING what is going on in its environment, but the mother's and father's attitudes and FEELING toward the pregnancy can have an impact as well. What a fetus experiences in the womb can create expectations, predispositions and vulnerabilities. A fetus doesn't have rational thinking. It doesn't know the terminology for the sensations that it is experiencing....but it FEELS them nonetheless.

The OFC (orbitofrontal cortex) of the brain is a part of the brain intricately tied to the limbic system. The limbic system is what governs our emotions. (you know, the THINGS we have been taught to suppress?) The OFC serves as the "control center" of our emotional lives. It interprets the nature and value of our environment. This is where the 'infancy period' of life is embedded. It is continuously evaluating the emotional significance of every interaction we encounter. This "evaluation" occurs in microseconds. It determines who "loves us" and who doesn't. Who is "safe" and who isnt. It goes even further and determines how MUCH we are loved and HOW safe we are.

One of the many ways the OFC affects us, is based on cues from pupillary reactions of those who care for us. Dilated pupils tend to indicate positive emotions…happy, enjoyment, affection, love. These interpretations are subconscious and happen almost instantly. The size of our parents' pupils when interacting with us had a PROFOUND impact on our brain formation. The formation of the brain then impacts our interpretation of these "indicating cues" in others later in life.

Every human being NEEDS a HEALTHY attachment connection for optimal development. An infant requires MORE than *someone to take care of it*. They REQUIRE an ATTACHMENT BOND.

When there is a dysfunctional attachment bond (particularly with parents or caregivers) this will adversely affect the brain during the infant period and ultimately it will negatively impact all future relationships with others. This also contributes to a poor relationship with SELF. The lack of this bond can only intensify the *mind body disconnect*.

Studies have shown high levels of adrenaline and cortisol in the mother's system can increase the child's susceptibility to emotional distress by affecting the child's autonomic nervous system. There are studies linking these chronically elevated hormones in the mother resulting in learning difficulties, behavioral problems and GI disorders in these children.

The bottom line? We were sensitive to the feelings our parents experienced during our gestation and then continued to download information from our parents, families, and environments intensely during the first 3 years of life and continued at a steady pace through age 7.

DNA is the "blueprint" for our existence. It determines the make-up of every cell and the hereditary traits of every person. The DNA of the cell is where our feelings and emotions are registered and recorded. (imprinted) This is called *cellular memory*. Each cell has an internal mini hard drive that this imprinted information is stored on. When our cells replicate, these suppressed feelings and emotions are encoded on the new cell. This "imprinting" governs our belief system and impacts our behavior, personality and responses through our life. Every cell in our body is impacted by our thoughts, feelings and emotions.

Many times we don't understand where our "trauma" developed. Our beliefs are established from the conclusion we draw from our *PERCEPTIONS*. And from our emotions associated with these perceptions. We don't allow the admission of any information that is inconsistent with our BELIEFS. It doesn't matter if these beliefs are real or not. TO US, they are REAL.

For example: If at birth, we perceive the feeling of "rejection." Maybe our mother was struggling emotionally, financially or relationally. She was worried about how she was going to care for us. SHe may have FELT stressed and panicked. She may not have been able to devote her time and affection to us due to other responsibilities (older children at home, work, caring for a parent,ect) Even though we don't know the WORD REJECTION, we just know that we FELT rejected. We may internalize this feeling and enter into life with this "belief". Our belief system is that 'being rejected' is our predestined path. It is the road of life on which we MUST travel. Once our subconscious mind establishes a belief, our conscious mind works to "prove it right." The intention of our mother was not to make us feel this way. She LOVED us dearly. It was our interpretation (our perception) that created self limiting belief.

'Feeling' will always win over 'thinking'. When these two things are not in agreement, there is inner conflict. Our distorted perspective will guide our interpretation to form a self belief that isn't accurate. But our interpretation makes it TRUE to us. Our EGO (mind) has to be right.

Whenever our mind determines a belief, our mind then works to "make it so". The mind will interpret things to confirm this belief. It can direct and create situations where these beliefs are fulfilled. Self limiting beliefs are detrimental to our growth and can interfere with relationships, careers, etc. Some examples of these beliefs are: *"I'm hard to love". "My feelings dont matter." "I have crappy genetics so I am destined to be ill"*, etc. These beliefs can be heavily impacted by inadequate attachment bonds.

Beliefs can shift biology. Your body can create its own pharmacy of chemicals and hormones to heal. It can activate/deactivate the immune system. Whatever you TRULY BELIEVE in this moment is giving directions to your immune system. You are either saying:

A. *Suppress and deactivate*   or   B. *Clean, repair and heal.*

If these beliefs are left unchanged, they become self-fulfilling prophecies. When the mind is validated, we get a sense of 'comfort'. No matter if the validation is self

imposed and not based on reality, or if it is
INCORRECT. We perceive a sense of *comfort and
control*. BOTH indicate we are right, and therefore; it
proves to re-confirm these inaccurate and limiting beliefs.

AWARENESS

Of our WORDS —>

One way our subconscious works to create our
environment is through our SPOKEN WORDS.
Emotions are energy. WORDS ARE ENERGY. They have
the power to hurt, harm, humiliate. They can tear people
down. Words can also HEAL. They can also build others
up. They can inspire.

*"I AM" are two of the MOST POWERFUL words we
can speak*. These words should be used with TRUE
INTENTION. They set things in motion. For example: "I
am unlovable". "I am never going to heal." "I am not able
to release these blocked emotions." These are words of
action or action phrases. You are stating a limiting belief
or perception as FACT and with conviction. It becomes
your TRUTH, even though it is FAR FROM TRUE.

"I HAVE" are also 2 words of power. These words
should be used with deliberate thought. When they
diagnosed me with Lupus, I would tell people my story

and it would contain the words... "I have Lupus." I am very diligent about this statement now. MY TRUTH is that I do not WANT this illness. I am bidding it adieu, I dont want it sticking around. I now say "When they diagnosed me with Lupus." Or, "The Dr has advised me that my labs indicate Lupus."

Words have power, and this power causes hormones to be released in thc body. If negative words have that kind of effect and power over the body, consider what effect POSITIVE WORDS will have! "I am lovable", "I am healing". "I am releasing these self limiting beliefs and emotions".

It is important that you develop an awareness for the words you speak. Words set in motion what you are manifesting in your life.

Of LISTENING —>
Listen to what you are saying TO AND ABOUT yourself... Your self talk. How do you speak to yourself? Are you harsh? Judgemental? Degrading? Demeaning? Do you speak gently? Are you kind and supportive? What tone do you use? Are you repeating things you heard as a child? Or things you FEEL about yourself?

The best way to test your self-talk is to imagine a 3-4 year old child in front of you. Would you speak to that child in the same manner you speak to yourself? If the answer is no.... Then STEP ONE is changing how you speak to yourself.

Initially it will be a slow process. You will catch yourself AFTER the fact more than you will BEFORE. However, over time this becomes easier.

Just like a child with a verbally abusive parent can't thrive..... A body with a harsh mind can't thrive.

The body doesn't know the difference between you talking harshly to yourself or someone else speaking harshly to you. If a loved one, coworker, or even a stranger spoke to you in a harsh way, it would result in an emotion that would impact every cell in your body. You will still experience the same response if YOU are speaking harshly to yourself. YOUR WORDS are the foundation of the healing process in your body.

Are you "claiming" your illness, or condition? "_MY cancer is stage 2._" By calling it YOURS, you are claiming it AS YOURS. You are telling the narrative from the victim perspective.

As I said before, I am diligent with my words now. The majority of the time, I will now say, "_I was diagnosed with_

Lupus" instead of "*I have Lupus.*" I don't WANT to have this condition, so I choose NOT to CLAIM IT.

Of our THOUGHTS —>
(Our FEELINGS)

By listening to your words and what you are saying to/about yourself, you can begin to understand your THOUGHTS.

You can begin to recognize your thought process and patterns. You will become familiar with your thought cycles. This will allow you to trace back to FEELINGS. Do you have a negative perspective? Are you always focusing on the negative? Do you look for ways for things to be YOUR FAULT? Do you always apologize even if it was something out of your control? Feelings are usually what trigger the thoughts. These 'feelings' also impact how you talk to yourself and the story you are telling.

Through our thought processes we find ourselves caught in a cycle that is detrimental to our health. Thinking creates feelings and feelings create thought. The more we think the same thoughts that cause us to feel a certain way, the more we become impacted by our thoughts.

Depending on what we are thinking and feeling, we are actually creating our state of BE-ing. What we think about and the energy with which we think it, directly impacts our health and the choices we make. For most people with Chronic illness, many of their thoughts DO NOT SERVE their health.

Our thought processes and cycles are often based on INCORRECT PERCEPTIONS and interpretations. This sets us up to continue to incorrectly perceive and interpret every event and situation from this vantage point. This is why we often feel validated and confirmed through our thoughts. As the quote goes: *We don't see things as they are, we see things as WE are.*

Gaining awareness of our thought patterns and cycles is instrumental to our healing process. Just because we have a thought DOES NOT MAKE IT TRUE.

These distorted thought patterns create an unhealthy view of reality, better known as, cognitive distortion, often leads to a life of depression, anxiety, relationship problems, and self-destructive beliefs and behaviors all of which over time, damages the body. Research by van der Kolk (2014) illustrates the profound impact of trauma (events/perception of events) on the body.

Now is the time for ACTION. Negative thinking results in a negative state of BE-ing. It's time to interrupt this pattern and step out of old routines and change your way of thinking. You will change your way of BE-ing.

Of our ACTIONS—>
There are many approaches to resetting your thought processes. One way is cognitive behavioral therapy (CBT), where you work with a therapist to identify faulty thought patterns and interpretations and practice techniques to help reshape these negative patterns.

Ways to become more aware of your thought patterns:
- *Awareness - Of your words and beliefs. Pay close attention to what and HOW you think.*
- *QUESTION - These thoughts or beliefs. Are they based on FACT or OPINION? Is there TRUE evidence to support these beliefs and patterns?*
- *Gather Evidence - Gather evidence for or against your thoughts, assumptions, and beliefs. Remember, cognitive distortions are biased and inaccurate. However, they are deeply embedded in our psyche. List the facts that show a belief is accurate, and compare these facts to a list that shows the same belief is distorted or incorrect.*
- *Resetting thought patterns - This requires resetting our incorrect and detrimental thoughts with ones*

that are rational and positive. In order to 'think differently' you have to replace the distorted interpretations and beliefs that have been embedded.

2.

Our "Self" Beliefs

(Limitations)

Our self-beliefs influence every aspect of our lives, from our relationships to our health. For me, these beliefs began forming in childhood and shaped how I saw myself for decades.

Change doesn't happen overnight, so please don't expect to correct a lifetime of limiting self beliefs in one session. This can take time, maybe even years. The focus is to understand WHAT you believe about yourself and WHY you believe this about yourself. Then to change these limiting beliefs that are not based on reality. They are based on words you may have heard, actions that you perceived, situations in which you survived, or from someone else's inability to communicate effectively.

It is time to recognize that your limiting self beliefs may be founded on incorrect perceptions, or false interpretations that have negatively impacted your SELF IMAGE and limited your growth and abilities/opportunities. Self-beliefs are the subconscious conclusions we draw about ourselves based on experiences and perceptions. They shape how we see the world, respond to challenges, and even affect our health.

I was the only girl on both sides of my family for 14 years. When I was little, I would go spend time with my *Nanny and Grandpa,* which were my mother's parents. My grandparents lived in a small trailer park. It was a community where everyone knew everyone. After dinner, it was customary for my Grandpa and I to take a walk around the park and visit with all of his neighbors. Each and every home we went to he would share my latest accomplishments. "*My Angel* had a school concert this month." "*My Angel* got all A's on her report card." He had a way of making simple events seem like monumental milestones. Don't get me wrong, He could be STERN if he needed to be. But, for the most part, I was put on a pedestal and treated like a china doll. As if I were the only girl ever to be born to a family. I was always made to feel special.

My father's family was a different story. Having had only boys. They took a different approach. Everything there hinged on treating me differently. "Don't make her cry, *she's a girl.* Don't roughhouse with her, *she's a girl.* Don't make her sweaty, *she's a girl.* Don't get her dirty, *she's a girl.*" My perception of those statements was that being a girl meant '*less than*'. It was something to be looked down on, it was a disappointment. (It wasn't until I was much older, and had started on my own journey of self discovery, that I came to learn these words had been meant to be positive in their own way. They were meant for my uncles to stop and take note that I was in fact, a girl and to treat me gently. However, that was NOT my perception at that time.)

This dynamic reflected not just family attitudes but also cultural expectations about gender, which I internalized as part of my identity. So I decided I was going to be the meanest, loudest, most aggressive, one in the bunch. I *would be* seen. I *would be* heard. I wouldn't just be '*a girl*', I would be the *toughest GIRL*!

This incorrect perception planted a seed of self-doubt, self-loathing, and lack of self-love. This inability to love myself effectively, instilled a limiting self belief that I was not as good as everyone else. This was a cage in which I put myself. I locked the door. And through the key as far away as I could. I went through life with this caged view. Limited by the walls I had put around me. By my incorrect perceptions and misinterpreted BELIEFS of myself and who I was.

It wasn't until a very dear friend of mine, who could see beyond MY LIMITING BELIEFS and my "tough exterior", found the key, opened the lock and swung open the cage door for me (Metaphorically speaking). They began to coax me out of the cage that I had claimed as 'my identity'. Slowly bit by bit, I began to venture out. First by their encouragement and guidance, and then by the spark they had inspired within me. I started to see myself differently. I started to FEEL differently. And.... I began to love myself.

Now, don't think this was easy. In the beginning, it was one step forward, three steps back for me. It can be very difficult to let go of self limiting beliefs. These early experiences shaped my self-talk, which over time became a cycle of negativity. Here's how I began to break free from that pattern.

My self-talk had always been extremely harsh. "You stupid idiot! You, moron! You don't deserve the air you breathe! How can you be so stupid?" These were common phrases (along with many more that were far more damaging) I would say these things to myself on a daily basis.

Studies show that negative self-talk can activate the stress response, leading to chronic health issues like anxiety and inflammation (Kross et al., 2014).

> *Our body does not know the difference between ME saying these things to myself or someone else saying them to me. My cells, my tissues, my body as a whole, responds in the same manner to this negativity no matter who is speaking the words.*

So imagine, living in a body that you have talked to horribly for over 40 years. How is that body going to thrive? Just like a child in an abusive home doesn't thrive, a body with an abusive mind will not thrive. At 43, my body was no longer thriving. And it was barely surviving.

I slowly began to become very aware of the words I chose to say. The names I called myself, the criticism, the negativity. I set a daily goal of sitting on the side of the bed every morning and saying five positive things about myself.

When you have lived in a negative mindset for the majority of your life, this seems almost impossible and in the beginning it felt very fake. I said very silly things like: "I like that I have brown eyes. I like that I have brown hair." I was stating facts, not opinions or beliefs. Over time the positive things became easier. "I have a kind heart. I am compassionate." Eventually I began to say *"I love myself. I am proud of the woman I have become."* Talk about a transformation!

I also began to focus on the words. I said to myself, when I would make a mistake, or do something that I interpreted to be wrong. *"Silly girl, you knew better than that." "All right.. now that we know that way doesn't work, we will try it again! You'll get it this time."* What I began to notice was how my body responded overall. I didn't feel the need to punch something or scream. In the past, after berating myself, I would always feel the need to do those things. My words would only add to my anger, hurt or frustrations. Usually inciting me to physically react... Slamming doors, kicking the air, stomping.

As I became easier on myself. I started to notice I was laughing at my mistakes, which was not something I would ever do when I messed up. This was a long process. And did not happen overnight. It took consistent effort to be aware of the way I talked to myself. It is still a work in progress, most days I am WINNING the battle, others, I have to apologize to myself and remember to allow myself grace and understanding.

I can clearly remember when the reality hit me of how my self-talk had changed. I had made a very big mistake.

One which resulted in a lot of effort to correct the matter. However, at the time, I simply said to myself " *that was a big one, kiddo! Did you mean to goof up like that? No you didn't. So don't beat yourself up, this is fixable. And yes, it appears to be a mess right now, but look for the lesson in the mess.*" This was not a phrase that would've ever been uttered *by myself to myself.* And for it to come out so effortlessly, was a wonderful realization of just how far I have come in my endeavors.

Once I felt like I had a good hand on my self-talk, the next step was to start understanding why I believed what I did about myself. Why did I believe I was unlovable? Why did I believe I wasn't good enough? It was time to tackle those self-limiting beliefs.

As of the writing of this book, I have come to understand AND CHANGE many of them. However, I still have many more to go. As I have said: healing is a process, not an end goal. With each step in the process, I have become wiser, stronger, faster, and more motivated to continue this journey!

Suppression vs Repression:

Suppression is when we force the information (feelings/events/etc) out of our awareness. We consciously *choose to not allow the thought, feeling or action even though we are aware of it.* Many times we suppress because we feel that "I just can't deal with that right now."

Repression, also known as *dis-associative amnesia*, is similar to suppression, except for, it involves *unconsciously blocking out unpleasant thoughts, feelings and impulses.* Sometimes we repress traumatic past memories because they are so upsetting.

An example of repression would be, a person having no recollection of the physical or sexual abuse suffered during childhood. Initially this saves the person from the intense negative emotions associated with these memories. However, these memories don't just disappear; they become lodged in the body where they eventually manifest through a symptom, or series of symptoms and may continue to influence our behavior.

Repression can contribute to anxiety, which starts when a traumatic memory threatens to enter the conscious mind. Freud believed repression to be the root of people's "neuroses," the term he assigned to the mental struggles such as stress, anxiety, and depression. He felt that repressed feelings and emotions, although subconscious, were still present and could resurface in disturbing forms. The inability to process and come to terms with repressed material could lead to psychological problems such as poor concentration, irritability, anxiety, insomnia, nightmares, and depression. He believed that maladaptive and destructive patterns of behavior such as anger and aggression could emerge due to triggers of the buried memories.

Emotional repression often relates to childhood experiences. If showing your feelings in childhood led to negative or 'hurtful' responses from those around you, it probably felt safer to avoid this behavior.

Adults with repressed emotions often feel out of touch or disconnected from their feelings and bodies. You usually continue to bury strong emotions without realizing what you're doing. For the most part, people tend to repress strong emotions, especially those associated with discomfort.

This includes emotions like:

anger

frustration

sadness

fear

Disappointment

Hurt

grief

Abandonment

These emotions are often described as negative. It's common to repress emotions you consider "bad". Those with repressed emotions often have trouble naming these emotions or any heavy emotion they are feeling.

Once you gain the awareness that you have repressed emotions, it is important that you begin practicing emotional expression.

Emotional repression may also restrict people's ability to connect with those in their life. It fosters an insensitivity to negative emotions, or an AVOIDANCE. It is also difficult for people to tolerate negative emotions of others or even being around those who are emotionally suffering. It can also affect a person's ability to be genuine and authentic in their relationships.

For many people, a situation that brings uncertainty triggers an unconscious protective measure that allows us to cope with unpleasant emotions. Coping mechanisms are strategies that help people deal with uncomfortable situations and emotions.

Coping mechanisms and defense mechanisms are terms that are often used interchangeably. To clarify, they are not the same. Coping mechanisms are skills a person uses intentionally to deal with stressful situations. Defense mechanisms are automatic unconscious strategies used to protect ourselves from anxious thoughts or feelings.

Emotional awareness is the first step where we identify and define what is underneath all the layers and to take control of our lives. It is recognising and understanding our emotions. Seeing them for what they are. We must become self-aware to recognize our emotions as they happen.

When we routinely employ our defense mechanisms, it interrupts our emotional processing. We may feel as if we are not 'really feeling' our emotions. (Disconnected) This interferes with our ability to work through issues. This is why it is important to become aware of your personal tendencies so you don't let your defense mechanisms overtake your emotional growth in life.

How do you handle stressful situations? Do you live in a state of denial when you receive bad news? Do you constantly excuse your behavior or the behavior of others? These are just a few common defense mechanism examples that can get in your way or impact your relationships if you aren't aware of them.

It is important that you understand some common types of defense mechanisms. These can range from shifting blame, to projecting, to shutting down emotionally. Each person has their own unique defense mechanisms. Only with practice do they become easier to recognize.

<u>Common Defense Mechanisms:</u>

1. Denial - When a situation or emotion becomes too much to handle, you may cope by refusing to experience it. By denying reality, you are essentially protecting yourself from having to face and deal with the unpleasant event and pain that accompany it.

(Denial and repression may seem similar on the surface. To clarify, denial involves the outright refusal to accept a given reality.)

2. Repression - Repression involves completely forgetting the experience. Your mind makes the decision to bury the memory in your subconscious. The goal is to prevent painful, traumatic or dangerous thoughts from entering

your awareness. *This is often the case with child abuse or other traumatic experiences.*

3. Regression - With this mechanism, you revert back to a childlike emotional state. Your unconscious fears and anxieties reappear causing you to revert to a younger level of development and in many cases, childish behaviors. This is done as a way of protecting yourself from confronting the actual situation. If during an argument with your spouse, you stomp off, slam the door and give your partner the silent treatment..... You are exhibiting regression. This mechanism shuts down communication and inhibits the ability of the relationship (*and the person exhibiting this mechanism*) to grow and evolve emotionally.

4. Avoidance - One of the MOST COMMON mechanisms. It is human nature to avoid uncomfortable situations or events. When we do this for too long, the issues we are 'avoiding' only tend to compile. People exhibiting an avoidance mechanism may appear to be resistant, defiant, or may procrastinate along with other traits.

5. Displacement - If you have ever had a stressful day at work, then come home and take it out on your loved ones? Then you have experienced

displacement. This is typical defense mechanism examples in busy adults. You're transferring your emotions from the person or situation that is the target of your frustration to someone or something else entirely. Subconsciously, you may believe that confronting the source of your feelings may be detrimental, so you shift the focus toward a target or situation that is less intimidating.

6. Projection - A common defense mechanism for avoiding unpleasant feelings. You may be in a situation where you feel uncomfortable or anxious. You perceive that others are staring at you with criticism or judgment. They do not say anything or do anything that is objectively negative, but your insecurity causes you to "project" your feelings onto others. This defense mechanism is one of the most damaging. It can foster heightened feelings of paranoia and anxiety. It also contributes to limiting beliefs about ourselves and others that cause you to become bitter, suspicious or distrustful.

7. Reaction formation - With this defense mechanism, you are behaving in a way that is opposite of which you think or feel. Where you replace an unwanted or anxiety-provoking

emotion with an opposite emotion and then express it in an exaggerated or dramatic way.

8. Rationalization - When you try to explain your bad behavior away, or to justify your behavior. You blame someone else for provoking you. Or make excuses for why you did/said what you did.

9. Sublimation - The defense mechanism where you transform your conflicted emotions, unmet needs or unacceptable impulses into productive channels. This is a POSITIVE defense mechanism and can help you progress emotionally.

10. Disassociation - This mechanism centers on escapism. It involves mentally separating yourself from your body (mind-body disconnect) to distance yourself from traumatic experiences. This is a common response to trauma. However, it creates separation from your true BE-ing.

Pay attention to the mechanisms you employ when you are in an emotional or stressful situation. Once you learn which mechanisms you often employ, it is time to take responsibility for your own emotions. You can begin to break those patterns and stop using defense mechanisms. Implementing modalities like mindfulness and healthy expression of your emotions and practicing envisioning your NEW SELF can help you shift your mindset and see your world in a more positive way. Changing our self-beliefs takes time, but each step forward is a victory. By transforming how we see ourselves, we lay the foundation for healing mind, body, and spirit.

3.

"Stress"

(What it is, what it DOES)

In chapter 1 we touched on stress. So let's take a deeper look.

Stress is often misunderstood as an emotional response, but it's far more than that. It affects every system in the body, especially when chronic.

HIGH FUNCTIONING stress and anxiety can mean the typical symptoms: *fear, worry, increased heart rate, difficulty sleeping, jumpy, or even spaced out.* However stress can also manifest as: *inability to relax, the need to ALWAYS be busy, working well under intense pressure, procrastination, taking on too much, irritability, mood swings, sleeping too much, intense dreams, jaw pain, chronic tension in neck and face, scattered thoughts, intrusive thoughts, OVERSPENDING, habitual shopping, hoarding, impulsive, indecisiveness, disorganization.* There are many ways stress and anxiety can manifest. The symptoms are not the same for everyone.

Stress is your body's response to any change—whether positive or negative—that demands attention. This response, when chronic, can disrupt physical and mental well-being.

As we have discussed, the body's response to most stress is fight or flight. The series of evolutionary responses in the body that make it ready to 'run away' or 'fight what is in front of it'.

When we stay in a prolonged state of stress, we get stuck in fight or flight. This impairs the body's ability to use the nutrients it ingests. It also burns up any energy stores the body may have. Long periods of stress exposure can set the stage for chronic disease.

For instance, chronic stress can impair digestion, leading to nutrient deficiencies and gut health issues like leaky gut syndrome. When normal amounts of stress occur, these hormones are released in response to the perceived threat and then fade away shortly after. Studies show chronic stress disrupts the balance of pro-inflammatory and anti-inflammatory cytokines, increasing the risk of autoimmune diseases (Cohen et al., 2012).

Anxiety is the mind and body's reaction to perceived stressful, dangerous, or unfamiliar situations. It's the sense of uneasiness, distress, or dread you feel before a significant event. Stress is not only an emotion, it is a physical response that affects many systems of the body. In short term situations, the effects are usually beneficial. However in long term situations (as in chronic stress) the effects can be damaging.

When our brain perceives a threat, Cortisol is released. If you need to outrun a predator this is the normal response of the body and therefore it is an efficient response. BUT, if you stay in this heightened state, your BODY perceives your kitten jumping up on the couch in the same manner as a predator. It can't differentiate between the two. THIS is when trouble can begin to occur.

Some of the prolonged effects of excessive cortisol in the body can result in *digestive issues, malabsorption, aging, sleep disturbances, weight gain or fluctuations, in ability to lose weight, and a suppressed immune response which can lead to frequent colds/flus or even autoimmune issues.*

Many factors determine how quickly your body recovers and heals. Your physical condition, the state of your immune system, pre-existing conditions, your immediate environment, all play a part...but STRESS is a major factor, if not the biggest contributor.

There are more studies than I can count on how stress impacts overall healing (and aging). On a cellular level, immunity is impaired and the chemical chain reaction needed for healing is interrupted. Prolonged levels of cortisol can result in systemic inflammation. Cortisol interferes with the production of anti-inflammatory substances called cytokines. This impedes the body's ability to heal. Persistent high levels of adrenaline can harm blood vessels, raise the blood pressure and adversely impact our cardiovascular health. Anxiety, worry and fear contribute to our mental load and increase the strain on our already taxed sympathetic nervous system. Cyclic negative thoughts keep us in a negative state and it becomes difficult to THINK or ENVISION ourselves as anything but ill. (Remember our discussion on thought patterns?)

Because we are stuck in flight or flight we are unable to digest our food adequately and therefore we don't absorb the nutrients from the food we eat. Actually we struggle to absorb any nutrients from food or supplements when we are stressed. This contributes to a decrease in energy production. Our energy reserves become depleted and the body begins craving carbs and high sugar foods because it feels 'energy starved.' Carbs provide short term energy, but because we have little to no energy reserves, we no longer have the desire to exercise or we feel poorly afterwards. We also tend to "overeat" carbs and therefore we tend to struggle with weight gain and elevated blood sugar.

Cortisol also impacts our reproductive system, growth processes, healing processes, and cognitive function. It affects the brain regions that control mood regulation, motivation and fear. High levels of stress hormones impair a person's ability to think clearly and logically, visual perception and often the ability to focus and pay attention. Cortisol also supports negative thought processes, which feeds our negative state of mind and body. Eventually, excessive exposure to high levels of cortisol can kill brain cells.

Adaptogens like ashwagandha help regulate cortisol, improving the body's response to chronic stress (Winston & Maimes, 2007). Herbal teas containing chamomile or lemon balm are calming and can promote relaxation. Incorporating things like breathwork, prayer and meditation can also reduce the effects of stress.

In today's world, it is almost impossible to not be "stressed". We carry one of the biggest contributors to our daily stress around in our hand most of the day. Our phone.

These devices, though extremely important at times, keep us in a constant state of alert. DING! BONG! Or some techno music or chime emits from them almost every minute. Even if we hit the silence button, we still feel the vibration or see the screen flash to let us know *YET AGAIN* that our attention is needed. MANY wear a watch so that in the off chance you miss the notification on your phone, you are sure to see the one attached to your wrist. It is hard to relax and find a state of calm when there is something constantly alerting you to a new text, email, sale ad or social media post. We are well trained to respond to "the ding". (When I was in grade school I remember watching a scientist that had trained a monkey to do a little dance every time he heard a specific bell ding..... Here we are 30+ years later, dancing like monkeys.)

Our constant connectivity through phones and social media amplifies stress, keeping us in a state of alertness that mirrors fight-or-flight mode. Prior to its introduction in our lives you rarely interacted with a large number of people. Social circles were limited to those around you. School, work, church, etc were our means of exposure. However, through social media, everyone interacts with everyone! We are constantly bombarded with pictures and posts of how AMAZING everyone else's life is! We begin to compare ourselves to others. Our homes, our lives, our kids, our jobs…. Everything is a competition. This can add an immense amount of stress for some people.

Others find stress in overstimulation. There are more streaming apps and movies than any one person can watch in their lifetime. Algorithms are created almost HOURLY to appeal to our every sense and need. We are at the mercy of a nameless, faceless, computer program that works to keep our attention and keep us stimulated and excited so we will *download, buy, click here, etc*!

Then there is LIFE and all the typical stresses it brings. You know, the "normal things" that have been around since the dawn of time! (Finances, death, divorce, jobs, family pressures, social engagements, school programs, athletics…the list goes on and on.) These are just SOME of the things that work together to keep us in a constant state of stress.

Then you take suppressed emotions into account – HEAVY WEIGHTS that keep us in a state of negativity. It can seem insurmountable, but it isn't! AWARENESS is the first step. Once you become aware you can now see things differently. You are no longer 'just functioning,' now you have a choice!

Wherever you focus your attention is where you also focus your energy.

The best way to move your energy away from disruptive stress and thought patterns is to change your focus.

We are always sending and receiving electromagnetic energy. Our body is constantly emitting a feeling, energy, or intention. Our thoughts and feelings create the electromagnetic field that surrounds our body.

Feelings are internal and part of our own consciousness. They dictate the way we perceive things. Emotions are external and linked to our thoughts, beliefs, past experiences, environment and so on. Each thought corresponds to a neural network of electrons that fire together and create electrical charges. The corresponding emotions create magnetic charges that emit a signal into our energy field. By combining what we think and what we feel we produce a state of being which generates an electromagnetic impression. And this impression influences our world.

To go a little further.....When it comes to daily happenings in our lives, the events themselves have minimal energetic effect on us. Our energy is more directly increased or depleted by the feelings and emotions we generate in our brains.

When you experience a positive emotion like gratitude or love, then your energy will elevate.. On the flip side, negative emotions (anger or grief) will drain your emotional reserves. Chronic negative emotions (anger, hate, resentment, grief) cause an energetic shutdown, which leads to depleted emotional energy and procrastination. Emotional energy is what impacts whether you feel happy or depressed. Your feelings are generated in your brain. They have nothing to do with the position you have at your job or your annual income. This is why some people who have very little material wealth are able to emit genuine happiness or joy and someone with a fat bank account may be severely depressed. It is about emotional energy reserves and whether you are being held down by heavy energy depleting emotions (chemicals) or lighter energy recharging emotions.

I had no idea why I felt like my batteries were ALWAYS near dead. I have struggled with this deep fatigue most of my life. When situations would arise that would demand an intense emotional response, I would be wiped out for days afterwards.

I was easily overwhelmed most of the time and dealt with severe anxiety which would lead to angry or disproportionate outbursts and responses. Please don't misunderstand.... My life hasn't been all dark! I have a good life and many wonderful experiences. In the past, had you asked me, I would have said I was "happy." But the weight of my heavier emotions had me at such a low level I couldn't really experience true happiness. The amount of anger and grief I was holding constantly drained me. It depleted me emotionally and energetically. My body couldn't withstand the chronic strain.

I had become so disconnected from my emotions and feelings that I couldn't FEEL that I was anxious. I no longer could FEEL the grief. I couldn't FEEL the other emotions associated with that loss: *anger, abandonment, fear*. Yet they were there. There and festering.

By recognizing the signs of stress and using tools to shift focus, we can break free from chronic stress and its damaging effects.

4.

MIND/BODY Connection

We can't be "present" in our body without our mind-body connection. I am a spirit, I have a mind and inhabit a physical body. The mind-body connection refers to the way our thoughts and emotions influence physical health. When we suppress emotions, the body often manifests them as pain, fatigue, or illness.

As I said earlier, we are 'trained' from birth to suppress our feelings. "Hush that crying up or I will give you something to cry about." This is the 'norm' for many people. We spend our childhood being trained and guided in what was and was not acceptable to express. Then we enter school and the training continues. Now we add teachers and peers into the mix. Then comes middle school, high school, sports, extracurriculars, dating, social settings. By now we have arrived at early adulthood and we are suppression experts. Many of us enter the workforce and the NEXT LEVEL of training begins....what is acceptable in society. We are now suppression and repression MASTERS!

It is not only taught in words but also in our environment and the interactions we have at an early age. (Birth to 3 years) There are other components that compound this "training".

Now that we have perfected our ability to suppress and hold in our emotions. We even have the confidence that we have ignored and swallowed them down so well that they are GONE! Never to be heard from again. However what we don't realize is that our emotions have not gone ANYWHERE except deep in our bodies and taken up residence. All of suppressing, ignoring, and swallowing emotions has set us up for a MIND-BODY disconnect.

Mind-Body Connection —>

Often when we are treated by conventional medicine, these areas, the mind and body, are treated individually. As if they were completely independent of each other. However, the conscious and subconscious relationship between the mind and body is an intertwining of physical health and mental health. When we suppress our emotions we are creating a disconnect of the mind and body. Our ability to FEEL and NAME our emotions is compromised. We may feel disconnected, detached, outside of our body or even numb just to name a few ways a mind-body disconnect may manifest. When dysfunctional attachment bonds are in place, these issues are even MORE exaggerated.

Depending on how long the emotion has been suppressed (or how deeply), you are likely not AWARE of what all is buried in the body. Studies show that emotional suppression can lead to dysregulation of the autonomic nervous system, contributing to conditions like hypertension, fatigue and chronic pain (Gerin et al., 2012).

> *Such was the case for me..... Remember what I said about being at the funeral home and seeing my grandpa. I could see him. But I couldn't feel him anymore. The pain was so overwhelming and devastating. I began pushing my feelings down thinking that "if I didn't love people, it wouldn't hurt me if this happened to anyone else." In that moment, I decided not to feel. That decision, born from grief, became the foundation of my mind-body disconnect.*

When they diagnosed me with Lupus, I was dumbfounded. I was unaware of any autoimmune issues in my immediate family. I am the type of person that needs to know WHY, HOW, WHEN, WHERE. I want to know the origin so I can understand what I am fighting. My subsequent lifestyle changes had gotten me 80% better but I KNEW there was more. I didn't know what, but I knew there was more.

Because I was still holding onto grief and anger, anytime I was 'triggered' such as being *upset, hurt, scared, sad, etc* the initial emotion that surfaced was always anger. Anger would rear her ugly head and wreak havoc on whatever situation prompted her to emerge. Over the years she had grown from an angry little monster to a large fire-breathing dragon that burned up everything in her path. Years of suppressed anger manifested as chronic inflammation and joint pain, reinforcing my need to address buried emotions.

It was during this time that I began working with a nurse who introduced me to essential oils. This friend had the inner strength and intuition to see my mind-body disconnect and lovingly but FIRMLY suggested I try a couple of essential oils. Being the (angry) skeptic I was, I was immediately resistant. She refused to allow me to detour from her efforts. She gave me Cedarwood and grapefruit oils. The essential oil cedarwood contains sesquiterpenes, which may calm the nervous system and promote emotional balance. I was instructed to put 3 drops of both oils on the bottom of each foot and back of my neck 2-3 times a day. I was also advised to deeply inhale the oils several times throughout the day. This was NOT APPEALING to me. I hated the smell of Cedarwood. It smelled like a litter box to me! And the grapefruit was just as unappealing.

After her absolute insistence, I decided I would use the oils for a month only to prove her wrong and that they wouldn't make a difference. And so every day I applied what I felt smelled like CAT PEE to my feet and the back of my neck. However, what I found after 4 weeks of consistent use (yes, I was committed and consistent to the applications) I began to feel a shift. I couldn't 'explain' the change I felt. The closest I can get is to say my mood was lighter. I was smiling more. I was having more emotionally 'good days' than bad. I decided to continue using the oils for another month, then another, then another.....and then I was hooked. I began diving into learning about oils, emotions, and how our trauma can impact us.

This is alo in the time frame that I came across the book, *FEELINGS BURIED ALIVE NEVER DIE by Karol Truman*. This book changed my life! I strongly encourage anyone who wants to come to a deeper understanding of themself to read it. At the end of reading the book, I decided to list every health issue I could ever recall having... Allergies, Hay Fever, Asthma, Colon issues and GI pain, Chronic Inflammation, lupus, etc. Using the illness reference in the book, I began to see that 'grief' or 'suppressed crying', was a recurring theme that was related to all the conditions I had listed.

This made absolutely NO SENSE to me at the time. I kept thinking "this is nonsense, I'm not grieving anything." I tossed the book aside and tried to forget about it. However it kept rolling around in the back of my mind.

It wasn't until something triggered a thought of my grandpa that I realized how badly it still hurt emotionally. I actually thought to myself, *this grief is killing me.* My thoughts circled back to the book. I decided to revisit the issue of grief. THIS TIME, I was more receptive and open minded. I began working through the grieving process, releasing the grief I had pent-up all those years. These emotions had been so suppressed I had no longer felt them. I couldn't feel much of anything except anger. Anger was ALWAYS there.

In focusing on grief, I came to realize I was still stuck. Remember, I said I consciously decided to not grieve, to not cry about it? Well here I was, 34 years later, realizing how my grief, my sadness, my anger, my refusal to cry had taken a toll on my body and now I was seeing it physically manifesting as systemic inflammation, Lupus, sinus and lung issues.

This awareness set in motion my ability to FINALLY begin working through the stages of grief and release of emotions. This began my mind/body "reconnection". I also implemented natural modalities like deep diaphragmatic breathing that can activate the parasympathetic nervous system, promoting relaxation. Gentle yoga or stretching to reconnect physical sensations with emotional awareness, and essential oils that I had researched for grief, sadness, and anger.

Oils affect not only our emotions, but physical conditions as well. I was also working with "the script" from *Feelings Buried Alive*. In a funny turn of events, as I continued to use Cedarwood and Grapefruit, I found a deep affection for those oils.... Cedarwood is probably my most favorite oil now. I love the smell, which for me, is strongly associated with liberation/freedom. It was the oil that started my emotional journey and was a foundational block in my emotional health.

What I have learned over the past 5 years, is that healing is an ongoing, never ending, process. We are more than just our diagnosis. And with the right guidance and information we can change the path we are on.

The Impact of "negative emotions" has an effect on the WHOLE. Imagine you are going fishing. You have your fishing pole and you attach several bobbers to it. One is Joy, one is Love, and the next bobber is happiness..... You also have sinkers on the same line. (*NOW- for all the fishermen out there, CALM DOWN.... This was a simple analogy! I dont put several sinkers and bobbers on my fishing line!!*) One sinker is anger, one sinker is fear, one sinker is resentment, another sinker is grief. When you cast your line, those sinkers (NEGATIVE EMOTIONS) pull your bobbers under water. They are below the surface and the sinkers take the line to the bottom of the lake. You still have Joy, Love and Happiness, but you can't really experience them to the fullest because the weight of the negative emotions is pulling them down.

As you begin to work on changing your mindset. You release grief and suddenly the grief sinker falls off..... What happens? The bobbers move closer to the surface.....maybe one pops up out of the water. You begin to release resentment..... The resentment sinker falls off. Another bobber breaks the surface. The weight of the negative emotions is losing its hold, and the positive emotions you were experiencing are now elevated. They are lighter, you can feel them more intensely. As the bobbers move on the surface of the water, you create a ripple effect and your "lighter, more positive emotions" can begin to impact others through these ripples.

When we are under the effects of negative emotions, we tend to think in a negative mindset. We PERCEIVE things from a negative perspective. We ruminate on negative thoughts and events. This 'negative state' becomes our "NORMAL". So if we receive a compliment, or hear something wonderful about ourselves, or are in a happy situation....we can't enjoy the FULL effect of these happy emotions because we are "under water".

This is another way to gain awareness of our state of mind and perspective. Many people are unable to receive a compliment. They will deflect, become embarrassed, or feel awkward. This is an indicator they are stuck in a negative state of BE-ing. Positivity is a foreign feeling to them. Even WORSE, some of them BELIEVE they are actually "positive people"!

Healing the mind-body connection requires intentionality. Tools like breathwork, mindfulness, and essential oils can help bridge this gap, allowing suppressed emotions to surface and heal.

Emotional blocks result in PHYSICAL blocks.

5.

Mind/Body and SPIRIT

The Physical:

Let's take a moment to discuss energy centers in the body. We have all heard the word 'chakra.' To some it is a positive word, to others it has a negative connotation. First, let me stress. I believe in the ONE TRUE GOD, His Son Jesus Christ and I believe in the Holy Spirit.

I also believe there is still MUCH we don't fully understand about the human body in reference to God. Moving forward, please note that the use of the term "energy centers" is in reference to specific points in the body that coincide with the endocrine system. I will also try to express how I have come to my OWN understanding of this concept and the perspective from which I operate regarding it.

The 'energy centers' are believed to transmit and receive energy at the seven levels in the body. Energy moves through the body via the nerves. Electrical impulses happen at the cellular level, and energy moves from cell to cell. This is how the Nervous System works.

The Nervous System, which is responsible for electrical communication, travels from the top of our heads to the ends of our toes. The Endocrine System is responsible for chemical communication throughout the body and it works very closely with the Nervous System. Hormones secreted from the endocrine glands are carried through the bloodstream to various organs and tissues of the body. There are seven main glands, and 7 main 'energy centers' that are located near major endocrine glands. These energy centers are known to transmit and receive energy at these glandular points.

The word "chakras" isn't mentioned in the Bible. But, we KNOW that God created our bodies with pathways for energy, electricity and chemicals to flow (nerves, blood, lymph, thoughts). He also could have created these energy centers throughout the body to receive and transmit energy messages.

We are a spirit and have a soul that resides in our body. The mind, body, and spirit are like three legs of a stool—each must be balanced to support overall health. In Genesis, God spoke everything into existence.

"And God said, "Let there be light": and there was light.

Before there was language, there was the Spirit of God. Through this same energy which moved upon the earth and waters, everything was formed, including mankind. The Bible tells us that God has not given us a spirit of fear, but of love, of power and a sound mind. These three spirits (love, power and sound mind) As I stated, each of the energy centers corresponds to an endocrine gland. They also are thought to correspond with a level of inner work to be done. Spiritual work.

When the priests and kings were anointed with oil in the bible, they were anointed beginning at the top of the head, and the oil would run down the rest of the body. This was VERY symbolic. When we look at each energy center and what it involves..... It makes sense to me that each center plays a role in our spiritual and emotional BE-ing as well as our physical.

1. Sound Mind (Crown)
2. Awareness / Wisdom (Pineal Center)
3. Communication (Throat Center)
4. Love (Heart Center)
5. Power and Strength (Solar Plexus Center)
6. Creativity and prosperity (Sacral Center)
7. Life and abundance (Root Center)

Again, These are MY beliefs based on my interpretations and readings, what I feel to be TRUE in my heart, and what makes sense to me from an anatomy standpoint. I do not follow other religions or thought processes when it comes to this topic. Especially when incorporating breathing into the process.

Some websites and books state that the 'root chakra' begins with the *kundalini spirit*. Many believe the Kundalini is an ancient energy present within our bodies. It is believed by some that the kundalini stems from the base of the spine and winds its way up to the top of the head, and is often described as a snake. Satan is often represented as a snake. I understand the hesitancy for some regarding these issues. I strongly encourage discernment in what you choose to believe. I do not follow the thought of kundalini. I am not in any way criticizing those who do, I just have my own beliefs and I apply those here.

I believe our LIFE FORCE comes from the breath of God. Genesis 2:7- *And the LORD God formed man of the dust of the ground, and breathed into his nostrils the breath of life; and man became a living soul. I believe every human being is alive through the breath of God.*

In Psalm 104:30- *The Spirit of God has made me, And the breath of the Almighty gives me life.*

If the breath of God can GIVE LIFE. It can also HEAL, can it not? This is my belief. I believe that if we incorporate the healing breath of God along with our awareness and self assessment then we can improve and heal our inner child as well as all of our broken parts. All of the disruptions and disconnects in our physical, spiritual, and emotional BE-ing.

Anytime I am meditating or working with a client, I imagine this bright energetic cord coming directly from God and into the top of my head. Much like a USB charger. I am "plugged in" to my source. It runs through me. There is no other influence that I entertain.

The Spiritual:

In my years as a nurse I have encountered MANY patients that struggle with the concept of "faith" and "God". I often hear questions such as *"if there is really a GOD, then why are children dying with cancer?"* This inquiry along with many others that have a similar amount of disbelief and anger (and no immediate answer) have been asked of me. Some at bedsides of those who are only acutely ill and will recover shortly. Others have been asked by those who are awaiting death's approach, are terminal and have no chance of recovery. ALL have left a mark on me in one way or another.

Unfortunately many of these people have experienced something in their formative years that made them feel violated or angered or abandoned. Their interpretation of the events led them to feel intense feelings that are easily directed toward the "old man in the sky" that they feel has abandoned them or 'allowed' these events to happen to them with no care or concern. Most verbalize comments like " *if there was a God, where was He when I was being beaten*?" Or some similar comment.

I don't profess to have any answers for WHY 'bad things' happen. What I DO BELIEVE is that to TRULY heal and restore the body, you HAVE TO HAVE a belief in a Higher Being. Without FAITH, there is NO HOPE. There is nothing to look forward to. There is just pain and agony for the living and then NOTHINGNESS after death. THIS MINDSET does not foster a healing state. IT CAN'T. How can the body HEAL if there is no HOPE, FAITH, GRATITUDE and LOVE. Afterall, these are some of the highest and most *'healing'* emotions that we can experience.

Those who are struggling with a disconnect of mind and body are also experiencing a disconnect with SPIRIT. This disconnect causes people to experience a "loss of SELF". This loss that creates a void, though often subconscious, leads people to search for something to fill it. Research shows that individuals with strong spiritual practices often report lower stress levels and better resilience to illness (Koenig et al., 2012).

If you are out of cell range, your phone will search continually for a tower to connect to, for a "signal". Our *spirit* will do the same. It is a necessary void, one that REQUIRES a connection. To deny it or refuse it will only leave you "continually searching" and with no "hope" in sight. This is a matter, of which, only YOU can decide. It is your SPIRIT that needs a connection. It is YOUR HEART that needs the healing that only a spiritual connection with a Higher Power can provide.

Most people believe that God is this overbearing and judgmental being that is looking for any and every reason to punish and destroy those who He chooses. At least this has been something I have heard many times through the years in direct patient care. God desires a relationship. Relationships require COMMUNICATION. You can talk directly to Him. Express your hurts and frustrations. Once you start a dialogue, the path will open up to you. There is no rush and no pressure. Move at the pace that feels right to you, in the MANNER that feels right to you. This is not a call for you to rush out and submerge yourself in a church. This is a call for something far more important! For you to submerge yourself in a conversation and relationship with God. The rest will work itself out in time. The most important thing is to establish a connection and to *accept that there is HOPE through FAITH.*

Again, I am not here to force anyone to follow my beliefs. I am simply saying that to restore your body, you will need to resolve your spiritual needs. This is a very personal and intimate internal evaluation. I encourage you to enter into this with the INTENTION of opening your MIND AND HEART to allow a relationship with the Higher Power.

Healing is a process of aligning the mind, body, and spirit. By embracing practices that nourish all three, we unlock the full potential of our well-being. Some ways to integrate mind, body, and spirit practices, such as:

- Mind: Journaling, cognitive reframing.
- Body: Yoga, breathwork, mindful movement.
- Spirit: Prayer, gratitude exercises, scripture study.

6.

So Why Don't We Heal?

(How beliefs impact outcome)

Healing is often elusive. Despite trying therapies, medications, or even making lifestyle changes, many of us feel stuck in a cycle of pain and frustration. True healing is more than physical recovery—it involves aligning the mind, body, and spirit

I've had many patients ask me why they aren't progressing, why they aren't healing? They will say *"I've changed my diet, I'm taking my supplements, I'm doing all the things I was told to do, why am I not feeling better?"* If you find yourself at this point it is important to ask some very thought-provoking questions.

Using a scale of 1 to 10, with 1 being the least, 10 being the best, ask the following questions: *(and be honest)*

1. *How much do I love myself?*
2. *DO I accept myself?*
3. *How WORTHY am I of recovery/healing?*

These three questions can give you a very good idea as to how you truly feel about yourself. Mental barriers often stem from self-limiting beliefs, like 'I don't deserve to heal' or 'I'm destined to be sick.' These thought patterns reinforce a state of illness and prevent progress. Identifying and reframing these beliefs is essential for healing.

It is extremely important that we focus on our self belief if we are to truly recover. As I have said before, a body with a harsh mind will not thrive. If we have harsh, self limiting beliefs, these will interfere with our healing process every time.

In working with clients, I will often ask on a scale of 1-10 (1 being the worst, 10 being the best) How much they LOVE themself. MOST will say, "oh, a 10 for SURE" and they will say it with CONVICTION. Most BELIEVE that they DO love themself more than they do. However the contrary is quite evident in the self-actions they take, the words they speak and the choices that they make on their journey. Many times, they are completely UNAWARE.

This is where the inner child meditation can be so effective, especially if we pull up our inner child, and find that we are not full of love for this child. If we view this child as obnoxious, a nuisance, unlovable, then, that is how we have been treating ourselves on a subconscious level. That is what we believe on a subconscious level: we believe we are not worthy of love, we believe we are a difficult person, we believe that we get in the way, we believe that it is our job to take care of everyone else, and put ourselves last, along with many other damaging self beliefs.

Some additional questions to explore:

Am I lovable?

Am I important?

Are my feelings as valid and important as those around me?

Am I good enough?

Can I be myself?

Maybe you grew up being compared to a sibling? Maybe you grew up and were expected to carry an adult load around the home? Maybe you had younger siblings and always felt the responsibility of caring for them? Maybe you made bad decisions or choices that resulted in someone being hurt? Maybe you found yourself in a regretful situation? Maybe you grew up on 'the wrong side of the tracks?' Maybe you didn't fit in with the popular crowd? Maybe you didn't fit in *with any crowd*? Any, and all of these can contribute to limiting self beliefs.

The perception of events, the actions, or the situation, resulted in a belief of yourself whether it was positive or negative. And this is the narrative we tell ourselves.

Over time, our limiting self beliefs along with high stress lifestyles, suppressed emotions, the daily go-go-go of American life, poor dietary choices, and unknown environmental/chemical exposures, our body may begin to manifest symptoms of dis – ease.

Healing begins within. It requires time, patience, and commitment to uncover the barriers that hold us back. Start by asking yourself: What belief or emotion am I holding onto that may be hindering my healing? Write it down, reflect on it, and begin the process of letting go.

We often turn to external solutions, like medications, supplements, or diets, expecting quick fixes. While these can be supportive, they rarely address the root causes of illness. True healing requires internal work—examining beliefs, emotions, and spiritual practices that support the body's natural processes. Healing happens in layers. For instance, addressing suppressed grief may reveal deeper issues of self-worth or fear. As we peel back these layers, we gain clarity and resilience, moving closer to wholeness.

This is when it is important to really dig, inward, and ask the hard questions. *Do I deserve to heal? Am I*

worthy of healing? Do I truly love myself? These deep
questions can allow us to begin to understand some of our
self beliefs: I am not good enough. I am not smart enough.
I am not handsome/pretty enough. I am unlovable.

I am none of these things!

For years I would tell people, "I am a difficult
personality and I am hard to love." This was NOT TRUE.
This was a self limiting belief I told myself frequently. I
understand now this was an attempt to protect myself
from feelings of rejection.

In the beginning these words impacted my ability to
heal. Since I was "hard to love" I obviously didn't *deserve*
to heal. This created a block for me for quite some time.
At least it did until I began to address my incorrect self
beliefs and learn to LOVE MYSELF. That is when my
beliefs started to change and my healing started to
improve.

I was *misinformed* about myself! I NOW
understand that <u>these beliefs </u>have been my limiting
factors, not the actions or events of my life. THESE
BELIEFS are what set the actions and events in motion.

I became determined to overcome these limiting
beliefs! I chose to open my mind, and see myself in a new
way. My old beliefs have only harmed me, my new

knowledge empowers me. I am worthy! I am valuable! I am important! I am the only me that this world will ever know and I will be the best version of me! I am worthy of forgiveness! I am worthy of a good life! I am worthy of healing!

Our thoughts are powerful. Negative beliefs, such as 'I'll never heal,' can create a cycle of despair, reinforcing physical symptoms. Cognitive reframing—challenging and replacing these beliefs with positive affirmations—can shift this cycle, allowing space for healing.

These beliefs are the '*poison in our pot*'. It doesn't matter how many healthy ingredients we put in the pot, if it has poison in it, it will not nourish.

<u>Ways to reset limiting self beliefs:</u>
- Identify your beliefs. (This may take time)
  Therapy is a great way to determine the limiting beliefs you need to address.
- Take responsibility. *We created these beliefs; you can do something about them.*
- Accept that your belief is INCORRECT
- Deconstruct this belief. *Examining what happened to create this limiting belief and how you interpreted what actually happened.*

- Take action! Replace your old truths with new ones. *THIS is where you begin to state your TRUTH!*
- Repeat the new "truth" back to yourself. *Do this often.*
- Surround yourself with people who support you. *This support system will foster reality. They will encourage your growth and be honest with you along the way.*
- Allow yourself to FEEL AND BELIEVE these truths!

Again, this is a PROCESS, not an end goal. Be patient, gentle and kind to yourself as you work on these things.

7.

MY Bread Crumb Trail...

(How To Start)

Healing isn't a straight path. It's more like a trail of breadcrumbs—small, seemingly disconnected moments that, when pieced together, create a map leading us toward wholeness. My journey began with frustration, evolved through trial and error, and eventually revealed the profound connection between my mind, body, and spirit.

I want to share the pivotal moments on my trail, not because I have all the answers, but because I hope they inspire you to reflect on your own. Each breadcrumb taught me something valuable and helped me move closer to a place of healing.

This was when I realized I had found the start of my *bread crumb trail*.....

The First Breadcrumb: Frustration and Seeking Answers

For years, I lived with chronic pain, fatigue, and a deep sense of frustration. I visited countless doctors, tried medications, and followed conventional advice, but nothing seemed to help. Each treatment felt like a temporary Band-Aid, and I was stuck in a cycle of pain and hopelessness.

The frustration became unbearable, and I realized I had two choices: accept that this was my life or take matters into my own hands. I chose the latter. That decision was the first breadcrumb, leading me to seek answers beyond traditional medicine. It wasn't an easy choice, but it marked the beginning of a journey that would change my life.

When I found the book that I had mentioned in previous chapters. *Feelings Buried Alive Never Die (Karol Truman)* and I decided to list all the chronic health issues I had dealt with from childhood to present. I also made a separate list with all the issues I had experienced over the past couple of years. I then referenced the back of the *"Feelings Buried Alive"* book and looked for the emotions and conditions listed under each health issue. I listed the major "health issues" that I had struggled with for most of my childhood and adult life. As well as my recent diagnosis of Lupus. What I found was a recurrence in certain "emotions and potential causes".

"Deep seeded GRIEF", "reliving childhood fears", "Chronic fear and anxiety" were the things that caught my attention. It was associated with autoimmune issues (LUPUS) and respiratory issues (Lungs)

"Laughing on the outside and crying on the inside" was associated with allergies and hayfever and autoimmune issues.

The GI issues and abdominal pain all had "holding on to old beliefs", "worry", "anxiety", "constricted energy flow".

These were a few of the "issues that I found may be a factor in my illness.

The steps I took involved the following:

A. Using the script in the book
B. Daily guided meditations for releasing suppressed emotions
C. Learning about and identifying unhealthy coping and defense mechanisms
D. NAMING MY FEELINGS!

Many people have no idea how important this is! When we suppress/repress, many times we are ignoring or avoiding what we are feeling. We don't "name it" so the body doesn't know WHAT TO DO WITH IT. It begins to store and compile this "unnamed feeling".

When we begin to work on our deeper emotions, it is important to NAME what you are feeling. "I feel hurt", "I feel betrayed", "I feel so ANGRY", "I am heartbroken, and sad over this."
Once we have identified the feeling, the body then realizes that all of this "unnamed stuff" sitting around and piling up is "hurt" or "betrayal", etc. It can now work to release these emotions from our body.

This is when you will learn to process a feeling.
"I am hurt."
The emotion I am currently experiencing is HURT. Once it has gained your awareness and been FELT, it may move on....it may persist for a little while. Heavier emotions such as grief, anger, sadness, etc may take longer to release. There is no TIME LIMIT for emotions to move on.
IF the feeling continues, it may require a deeper investigation. "WHY am I so hurt over these actions? What about this situation is the most

*hurtful?" Many times the next emotion will
surface. "I am so hurt because she betrayed me with
her actions. I feel betrayed."*

*This is usually when you realize hurt has lightened
up or may even cease to bother you.....now you feel
the emotion "betrayal." This is the next issue to
address.*
*You will continue this process until you no longer
feel the flood of emotions. You may go through a list
of 5 or 6, or you may only have one at a time. Once
you have named the emotion, allowing the body to
FEEL it without trying to avoid or ignore it, it will
begin to dissipate or diminish.*
This is step one of releasing emotions.

The Second Breadcrumb: Applying a Functional Approach

My perspective on healing shifted dramatically when I
started working in a functional medicine practice. For the
first time, I was introduced to the idea that symptoms are
not isolated problems but signals of deeper imbalances in
the body. This approach resonated with me, and I began
to see my body as an interconnected system rather than a
collection of unrelated issues.

One of my earliest breakthroughs came from addressing gut health. I eliminated inflammatory foods like sugar and processed grains and focused on nourishing my body with whole, nutrient-dense foods. Within weeks, my joint pain decreased by half, and my energy levels improved. This breadcrumb taught me that healing starts with supporting the body's natural processes, and it gave me hope that recovery was possible.

The Third Breadcrumb: Confronting My Emotions

While dietary changes and supplements helped my physical symptoms, I quickly realized that healing wasn't just about the body. I had spent years suppressing grief, anger, and fear, unaware of how much these emotions were weighing me down. They showed up in my body as tension, inflammation, and exhaustion, silently sabotaging my progress.

Confronting my emotions was the hardest but most rewarding part of my journey. Through journaling, breathwork, and essential oils, I began to process and release feelings I had buried for decades. I began to research which essential oils worked best for each emotion:

- Grief: Clary sage, Bergamot, Lavender.

- Anger: Cedarwood, Lavender, Ylang Ylang.
- Anxiety: Lavender, Lemon, Roman Chamomile were used.

I applied 2-4 drops of each oil to the bottom of each foot, as well as on the back of my neck and inhaled them EVERY DAY. It takes consistent use of essential oils over 3-4 months for them to create a cellular shift.

Oils are best used by applying to the soles of the feet, palms of the hands, or inhaled directly either from the bottle or from applying 2-3 drops to your hands and rubbing them together and creating a pocket over the nose to inhale deeply for 4-5 breaths. You can also apply oils to your hands and then run them through your hair. Spray a light mist of them over your pillow, or diffuse them directly over the head of the bed while you are sleeping at night.

I enrolled in an aromatherapy course so I could better understand and use the oils.... That is when my awareness and understanding took off. The introduction of essential oils and the way they can work on more than one issue and more than one EMOTION allowed me to heal exponentially faster than I had previously experienced.

I am not a fan of taking medication. I take supplements as recommended and when they are required. However, I have found that the natural effects of essential oils are very effective and are without the sensitivity or side effects of medications or supplements. One oil can address SEVERAL emotions in a subtle way that allows the body to transition into a higher level of health. Oils also can help with the physical symptoms of illness as well as regulate certain processes in the body over time.

The Fourth Breadcrumb: Reconnecting with My Spirit

The final and most transformative breadcrumb was rediscovering my spirituality. I had always believed in God, but during the years of pain and frustration, my faith had taken a backseat. Healing my body and processing my emotions brought me back to my spirit, reminding me that I wasn't on this journey alone.

Prayer became my anchor during moments of doubt. It wasn't about asking for instant healing but about finding strength and surrendering to a greater purpose. I also began practicing gratitude, focusing on small victories instead of the setbacks. Reconnecting with my spirit gave my healing journey meaning and grounded me in the belief that every step, no matter how small, mattered.

I strongly encourage you to reconnect with YOUR spirit. Implementing essential oils can help. I also recommend that you find a certified aromatherapist to work with on your health journey. When blended and used correctly you can benefit greatly from these modalities. I also believe to get the BEST RESULTS from essential oils is to use them with intention and prayer.

Prayer will enhance any meditation and treatment that you employ. My goal was not to script a "prayer" for YOU. I believe all prayer is very personal and needs to come from the HEART in reverence and humbleness. I believe it should be INTENTIONAL and from a place of personal DESIRE.

> *(Psalms 104:34 May my meditation be pleasing to him, as I rejoice in the LORD. <u>Isaiah 41:10</u> "So do not fear, for I am with you; do not be dismayed, for I am your God. I will strengthen you and help you; I will uphold you with my righteous right hand.")*

****

Dear Lord (Heavenly Father),
Forgive my misperceptions, incorrect assumptions and limiting beliefs that have contributed to my current feelings/thoughts/beliefs.

Please forgive me as I forgive others for the role I have assigned to them. Forgive me for the blame I have placed on You.

Help me to forgive MYSELF for any blame I have assigned to myself.

I ask that I be gifted discernment so that I may have ears to HEAR, eyes to SEE, a brain to UNDERSTAND and a heart to BELIEVE the TRUTH.

I ask for new awareness. Strengthen my mind, body and spirit connection so that I may live and 'BE' in the present. Fill my BE-ing with peace of mind so that I may be a light to others.

I ask that You please locate where this feeling/thought/belief of _________________________________ is hiding/stored in my body.

I am aware that incorrect mind, body and spiritual beliefs, thoughts, and feelings have contributed to this blockage. I ask that these beliefs/thoughts/feelings be removed from my mind and body and it be filled with Your truth.

I ask that you provide a reconnection of the emotional, energetic and spiritual pathways in my body so that I may begin to know and FEEL my emotions. Allow me to touch the hem of the garment.

Again, I strongly recommend that you apply your OWN prayer. However if this is a new concept for you, use the above as a template or a starting point.

You may have lived in a disconnected state for so long you can't REMEMBER what living in a 'emotionally feeling' body is like. It can seem strange and unfamiliar in the beginning. As you begin to recover from trauma, the good news is, it takes no time at all to acclimate to this state of BE-ing.

You will begin to realize that your mind is clearer. Your thoughts are easier to navigate. You are able to think more analytically. Your brain fog will begin to lift. You will become more aware of your 'triggers' and where you hold anxiety, stress and tension in the body. You will begin to FEEL your emotions instead of burying them or avoiding them.

It becomes easier to recognize when you NEED an emotional release and when (and where) you are 'holding' onto baggage. As you progress you will become aware of 'new wounds' that need addressed as well as 'old wounds' that need attention. You will become more aware of your own toxic patterns and negative defense mechanisms. This awareness will aid you in changing how you respond to events, circumstances or situations. These changes will positively impact your healing process. You will begin to CRAVE healing and self discovery.

As you learn to LISTEN to your body. You will begin to focus on INNER PEACE. With all of this knowledge and self awareness you will begin to UNDERSTAND your journey and you will learn the importance of forgiveness. (of yourself and others)

****

Sitting in the Doctor's office at 43, I knew my current level of HEALTH was a strong indicator that if I didn't make some serious changes, AND SOON, I would only continue to decline. I was TOO YOUNG for these problems! It was too young to hurt constantly. For my joints and muscles to ache like I was 90 yrs old, or needing to use my inhaler 8-10 times a day.

I determined that I needed to start at the BASE of my conditions. WHY Lupus? Why chronic allergies? Why were my lungs so compromised? Why did I seem to pick up every respiratory illness coming and going? But.......where did I begin? As my friend always says *"when the student is ready the teacher will appear*", well......I was ready. Let the lessons begin.

****

As I said earlier, I didn't realize I was carrying grief! I didn't know that it was impacting my body. If I DIDN'T KNOW, then how in the world was I going to release it? I got so frustrated when people around me would say "You need to release your emotions." I KNOW I DO.....but HOW? How do you release what you DON'T FEEL? How do you release something in your subconscious? What I found is that it's not as hard as one would think.

Once you determine what the issue is that you're dealing with, you can begin to focus on releasing it. In many instances, we have avoided this emotion/feeling for so long we've become numb to it.

First and foremost, you have to set the intent to release the suppressed emotions. You have to have a deep desire to release and heal. When I set out on my own journey, the first emotion I needed to tackle was grief. However, I didn't *feel grief.*

Because I didn't actively FEEL this emotion, I took a subtle approach to addressing it. I began using essential oils that worked well for grief. I applied them daily. I inhaled them frequently throughout the day. Oils need to be used with intention and commitment. Consistency is the key in having success with this approach. It can take 3-6 months of consistent use to feel a shift.

I also looked up, guided meditations for releasing suppressed emotions. (My ability to calm and focus my mind was minimal in the beginning) I started with 10 or 15 minute meditations. Initially I was always focusing on grief. The first couple of weeks I really felt nothing. But with persistence, I began to have small breakthroughs. There were a couple of times after the guided meditations I would find myself crying for small periods of time. Slowly, my body began to wake up to some of the feelings that were inside of it. As I continued, other emotions surfaced. Sometimes I would simply wake up, irritable, anxious, agitated, with no known reason. This became an indicator that I needed to spend time meditating.

When we are little, up to the age of three, we often don't have words for the emotions that we experience. We just know the feeling that we have. When the body doesn't know the name for something, it simply puts it somewhere in the body to be dealt with later. (It stores it in the warehouse of the body) If it is never dealt with, or we continue to avoid it, that emotion can take root and grow into a very ugly disease over time. As we become more in tune with our emotions, it is important to name what we feel.

When a feeling (emotion) is given a name, the body then knows whether to keep it or begin the release of it. Maybe as an infant, we struggled with a lot of hurts, or fears, or neglect.... As these things surface later on, and we state what that feeling is, "I feel and have felt hurt by you", "I feel, and have felt neglected in my life", "I feel, and have felt unworthy in my life", the body then knows the NAME of all these nameless emotions that have been stored within the body and that they do not need to be retained.

After naming the emotion, the next step is simply to allow the body to feel it. It may be for a few minutes, it may be for a couple of hours/days, it may be much longer. The problem arises when we try to suppress or avoid feeling our emotions. Once the body has fully 'experienced' this emotion, it will begin to lessen or dissipate until it has moved on. If you find that it hasn't, the next step is to investigate a little more. "I am so hurt." "He really hurt my feelings." "Why am I so hurt over this?" "Why did his actions hurt me so deeply?" *Because I feel betrayed.*"

What you may notice then, is suddenly hurt has moved on, and now betrayal has taken front and center.

BETRAYAL is the next emotion to work on. There can be many emotions tied to one event. Some of these emotions will demand immediate attention, others may surface overtime. I understand that working with our emotions can feel awkward, unfamiliar, or even painful. Unfortunately, there is no rushing this process. Rushing cuts short our ability to fully release.

You don't want to get "stuck" on an emotion. Ruminating over the event, replaying it over and over, is not therapeutic. It just creates an over abundance of the hormones and chemicals associated with those negative feelings. Now you are flooding your system with these negative feelings which are harmful, and can impact your mind and mood significantly. It is important when you investigate your emotions, that you don't get caught up in replaying the event(s).

Some of the hardest emotions to release:

Anger

Resentment

Rage

Hatred

Unforgiveness

Many of these emotions are the result of someone doing something to us. Sometimes it was unintentional, but many times it was very intentional. *Such as child abuse, sexual assault and many others.* It is important to understand that forgiveness is not condoning or dismissing what was done. Forgiveness is freeing your body from the emotion of *unforgiveness*, and all that is associated with it.

> *For example, if you and I were to have an argument in which you said something that made me very angry. We part ways and I walk around replaying this conversation and thinking how much I despise you, how angry I am at you, how much I hate you, or whatever thoughts I may have. These thoughts ruminate over and over. These negative emotions of anger, rage, hatred all percolate and fester inside of ME....*
> *As for YOU... You go on about your day, and your life. You have little to no regard for how these emotions/feelings are impacting me as I replayed this conversation over and over. You are untouched by my anger. You are untouched by my hatred and rage. You are oblivious to what it is doing inside of my body. You continue on with your life and no*

amount of my negative emotion is going to physically impact you.

However, I am suffering with physical ailments. I am suffering with negativity. I am allowing your words and actions to impact my every thought. Slowly these cyclic thoughts make me sicker and sicker. In essence, this event is continuing to traumatize me over and over and sadly it is being done by my own mind.

Forgiveness does not condone what was done. It does not excuse it. It does not "let them off the hook!" Forgiveness allows your body to stop traumatizing itself over what was done and it allows you to begin healing.

Unforgiveness is a punishment we impose on our SELF, because we are unable to impose it on the person that we feel deserves it.

I will be honest, I had heard many many times that forgiveness is more for me than the other person. I truly could not comprehend that statement. In my mind *forgiveness* meant that they were getting by with what they did. I have come to realize that is not the case. If a person is living and operating from a state of energy that is sowing pain, hurt and destruction (whether KNOWINGLY OR UNKNOWINGLY) eventually, they will REAP the fruits of that state. *A body cannot thrive in a negative state.* Those behaviors are of a negative energy. *They are also infectious.* That negative state will result in behaviors by this individual that are perceived as traumatic by those it impacts. Therefore, the seed of NEGATIVITY (in the form of anger, hatred, or unforgiveness) is sowed in anyone that this negative behavior affects. It is stored in the body of the offended and over time it may begin to grow/fester/rot. The only way to escape its effects, is to learn how to RELEASE. To forgive. To rise above that negative energy state.

If you don't, the virus of negativity invades, and in many ways it will use you to continue to spread. Just like a cold or flu. Maybe not in the same way as was experienced by you... (physical or emotional abuse) but it will continue through negative coping mechanisms and defense mechanisms. As I said, negativity is an "emotional virus" and it is VERY CONTAGIOUS.

I have heard so many people say, *"I understand everything you have said but you don't realize just HOW SEVERE MY ABUSE WAS! I CAN'T AND WON'T FORGIVE. THEY NEED TO KNOW!* They need to be held accountable and made to pay!" I AGREE! However, "payment" shouldn't come at the expense of YOUR HEALTH! I have spoken with many people who have worked through their pain to release their harbored emotions. Once they felt they had reached a level of FORGIVENESS, they were able to seek closure. Some have written letters to their offenders. Others have gone to the cemetery to speak from the heart. There were a few that chose to seek legal action now that they were not operating from a fear or terror of their perpetrator. Some have gone to face whoever violated them. They were able to do so from a place of peace and calm. They went to speak up for themselves NOW, because they hadn't been able to then. NOT to rectify or reconcile, but to be able to stand up for themselves and let their offender know that their negativity no longer had a hold on them. Many have walked away from that meeting and have not thought much more about that person and the pain they inflicted. Some continue to work on releasing the pain and emotions that may continue to surface associated with the trauma or event.

Your Trail Awaits

Emotions are something we will ALWAYS experience and at times need to address. However as you release the suppressed emotions it becomes easier to navigate the healing process. We all have a trail of breadcrumbs waiting to be uncovered. They may be subtle—a recurring thought, a deep intuition, or even a persistent frustration—but they are there, guiding you toward wholeness. Healing isn't about finding the perfect solution; it's about trusting the process and embracing each step, no matter how small.

Healing isn't a straight path—it's a trail of breadcrumbs, each leading you closer to understanding yourself. I hope my story inspires you to embrace the process and trust that each step matters.

8.

Reclaiming My Life

(Steps and Mediations)

In a world that glorifies multitasking and constant productivity, being present often feels like a luxury we can't afford. Yet, I've discovered that presence isn't just a gift—it's a necessity for healing. When we are fully present, we create space to listen to our bodies, process our emotions, and connect with our spirit. Presence is where healing begins.

The Distraction Trap

For years, I lived on autopilot. My days were filled with distractions: work, obligations, endless to-do lists. I told myself I didn't have time to slow down. But the truth was, I was afraid of what I might find if I stopped. My body was screaming for attention—pain, fatigue, and stress were constant companions—but I kept pushing forward, numbing myself with busyness.

Looking back, I see how this constant state of distraction prevented me from truly healing. How could I listen to my body or nurture my spirit when I was too busy to even sit still? Distractions became a way to avoid the discomfort of confronting my reality. But avoiding discomfort came at a cost—my health, my peace, and my connection to myself.

The turning point came when I realized that healing required my full attention. I couldn't keep running from my body's messages or suppressing my emotions. I needed to stop, breathe, and be present.

Being present isn't just about mindfulness or meditation—it's about truly experiencing life in the moment. It's about feeling the pain without numbing it, celebrating small victories without dismissing them, and listening to your body without judgment.

When I started my journey, I had very little guidance on HOW to navigate the world of releasing emotions. How was I going to succeed? I wasn't truly experiencing my emotions. I read as many books, watched podcasts, and listened to the "Masters" in this area.

I felt as if I was 'feeling my way through the dark.' I learned as I went and much of it was trial and error. My goal is to create an easy to follow outline of items for you to research and implement on your own journey. Use what

resonates, passover what does not. Reflect back often....
Just because something doesn't click today doesn't mean
that it won't somewhere down the road. Much of my
journey was going back to modalities and therapies that
didn't "fit" when I initially encountered them.

I intentionally left out the conventional treatments.
These will be the things your primary care doctor will
recommend and it is not my place to mention them here.

Remember, It is important that you do what YOU feel
is right for you....after all this is YOUR JOURNEY.

1. <u>Awareness</u>

    This is the first step to the healing process.
    Becoming aware that you need to HEAL allows
    your body to begin FEELING your emotions.
    Becoming aware of your emotions, self-limiting
    beliefs, defense and coping mechanisms and
    limiting thought processes are imperative to
    changing and healing yourself. Set your intention
    to begin FEELING and experiencing your
    emotions instead of shutting them down, refusing
    to feel them, or ignoring them.
    - Defense Mechanisms - Become aware of
      the defense mechanisms you employ.

- Coping Mechanisms - How do you handle emotional/situational issues? Implement a conscious effort to resolve these things productively.

2. <u>Self Assessment</u> - Become attuned to your body, your feelings, and where/how you hold tension is an important part of healing. Once you are aware of WHAT and WHERE you will be able to begin to change your negative responses and improve your communication as well as your mindset.
   - Focus on how you hold each emotion in your body. (Where you FEEL it) What does it make you experience? (Anxiety, GI issues, stiff neck, headaches, etc)

3. <u>Words</u> - Words have power. Become mindful and intentional with the words you speak. Our spoken words impact our thoughts, our emotions, and our behavior as well as every system in the body.

   Research indicates that when you speak positive words, it can positively impact your immune system, your brain, and your endocrine system. The same can be said for negative words, they will have a negative impact on these things.

Your body doesn't know the difference in You saying these things to yourself, or someone saying them to you. The internal response is much the same. Be intent with your words.

This applies to the way we refer to any 'dis-ease' we may be working to combat. Many times we CLAIM our illness as our own. If you noticed in the beginning of the book I stated *"I was diagnosed with Lupus."* I often will say "they told me, my labs showed Lupus" or "The doctors say my labs indicate Lupus." I never want to say "my illness" or "my lupus;" this implies ownership. I do not want to OWN this condition. Being intentional and mindful of our words is very important.

- Self Talk - Focus on changing your self talk to reflect a kinder and gentler tone. Speak to yourself as if you were talking to a 3-4 year old child. BE LOVING.
- We can also affect each other with our words. *Positive words can calm you or boost your immune system. However, negative and hateful words can cause your brain to perceive a threat and flood your bloodstream with hormones, which impact*

your immune system as well as your energy reserves.

4. <u>Thoughts</u> - Your thoughts are powerful! Use them to help you create the best version of yourself you can imagine.
   - Visualize what you want to obtain and how you want to feel. *See yourself already in possession of the healing.* Whatever you can imagine, you can become. Take time each day to visualize yourself healed, happy, and joyful.
   - When we connect our positive thoughts with high frequency feelings (happiness, joy, love, peace, bliss), we raise our overall vibration, and this is when healing occurs. Pay close attention to your thoughts. When you find they are negative, reframe them to something positive.
     - Think lovingly about yourself. Your thoughts are just as impactful on your physical health as your THOUGHTS.
     - Again, without a Higher Power, there is no FAITH, no HOPE.

Without Faith and Hope it can be difficult to have a positive mindset.

5. <u>Faith, Hope and SPIRIT</u> - We must come to understand that there is a HIGHER POWER than ourselves. FAITH in a Higher Power is a step in restoring our body. Faith gives us HOPE. It is heavily involved in the healing process. Make a decision to turn your life over to the guidance of GOD as you understand Him.
   - Faith restores our SPIRIT.
   - SEEK OUT KNOWLEDGE, DEEPER UNDERSTANDING and A CONNECTION with GOD. This will prove to fill the internal void of your spirit.

6. <u>Prayer</u> - It will strengthen your relationship with GOD and will allow you to develop a deeper conscious connection that empowers you. Prayer decreases the fight or flight response and triggers the release of feel-good chemicals in the brain.
   - Prayer can reverse brain damage caused by toxic thoughts and negative mindset.

7. <u>Meditation</u> - Develop a Meditation practice. This will positively impact your mind and increase awareness. It can also affect how you perceive and respond to the world around you.
    o   The benefits of meditation include better focus and concentration, improved self-awareness and self-esteem, lower levels of stress and anxiety, and enhance a positive mindset.

8. <u>Breathwork -</u> This practice activates the parasympathetic nervous system, reducing cortisol levels and calming the body's stress response—a key factor in creating an environment where healing can occur.

9. <u>Emotional Expression</u> -This is the acknowledgement and expressing of the emotions we were created to feel. Healthy expression allows us to understand the emotions, feel them and move them on.
    o   When we don't address emotions, we don't name them. The body doesn't know what to do with something that has no name. It stores these unnamed emotions somewhere

in the body. THESE emotional chemicals STAY in the body.

- By NAMING what we feel, the body now KNOWS what the emotion is and it no longer has any power over us.
- This action also strengthens the mind/body connection. The mind and body can now determine what we are feeling. NOW the body knows what these previously unnamed feelings were and can allow them to be FELT and processed.
- Name the emotion(s) - A name (or identity) is a powerful thing. It is a descriptor that allows people to make an assessment, a judgment and provide understanding of what you are dealing with.
  - Emotional self assessment. Ask yourself how you feel right now. Use "I" statements. "I feel hurt. I feel nervous. I feel angry."
  - Focus on the positive. It might not seem easy to name and embrace positive emotions at first. A body that has existed in a repressed or

negative state will feel AWKWARD and unfamiliar when it begins to allow emotions to be felt. Especially positive emotions.
  - Let go of self judgment. DO NOT judge yourself or tell yourself you shouldn't feel a certain way. Instead, validate the feeling: "I feel angry because his comments about me were incorrect and hurtful."

10. <u>Feel the emotion(s)</u> - Emotions have different weights. Some are very very heavy, others are light. If your best friend calls with the news "I am getting married!" You are full of happiness and joy. You are light and upbeat. This is a POSITIVE feeling and has a lightness to it.

    However, if your friend calls with news that she received a diagnosis of cancer, you experience a HEAVY emotion such as grief, sadness, or even anger. This can "weigh on you".
    - Heavy emotions can take longer to process and release. There is NO TIMELINE for processing. Heavy emotions must be allowed to be felt, experienced and then they will pass in their own time.

- This doesn't mean you should ruminate or wallow in these negative emotions, allow your body to feel and process but not to percolate in them. It is important that you don't force these feelings away or 'shut them down' either.

11. <u>Lifestyle Changes</u> - Do what you can, as you can. Every step forward is a step in the right direction. Physical improvements accompanied by lifestyle changes are SUSTAINABLE, these are changes that tend to last.

12. <u>FOOD is medicine -</u> Are you eating for nourishment? Or are you eating to feed a diseased state? Avoid if you can, but at the very least MINIMIZE the preservatives, processed foods, refined sugars, excess carbs that you eat. These are things that feed the disease process.
    - Eat the rainbow. Implement as many fresh fruits and vegetables as you can into each meal. (Veggie to fruit ratio 3:1)
    - Salads can be an expression of vitality. Get creative: Add berries,

seeds, nuts, different greens....
Experiment with dressings but
avoid the sugar laden concoctions
that pollute every shelf. Lean
towards vinaigrettes, oils, and
various seasonings.

13. <u>Supplementation</u> - The Liver and Lymphatic
systems need to function optimally for the body to
be able to detox and flush pathogens, toxins and
excessive emotions effectively.
    ○ Find a SUPPORTIVE physician or
      Naturopath provider and talk with them
      about supplements that support systemic
      detox and lymphatic drainage.
    ○ Have your Vitamin D levels checked 2-3
      times a year. Many people need
      supplementation and are unaware.
    ○ A good daily multivitamin is important
    ○ Collagen (preferably with amino acids) is a
      great addition

14. <u>Hydrate</u>-It is important that you flush your
system. You need to consume a minimum of 32-64
ounces of WATER daily.

- I often hear people tell me that they drink 6-8 cups of coffee a day so they are well hydrated. False. Caffeine causes cellular dehydration.
- Cellular dehydration is the root cause of nearly all disease, including cardiovascular disease and cancer.
  - Coffee and Sodas and Energy drinks are among the highest offenders in this arena.
    - The American Heart Association has stated that a 12-ounce can of regular soda contains as many teaspoons of added sugar. (+12 tsp)
    - Energy drinks can contain between 10-14 tsps of sugar per can.
- TEA - green tea, black tea, and herbal teas play a significant role in both physical and emotional healing. These teas, rich in antioxidants, polyphenols, and natural compounds, offer a holistic approach to

healing that aligns with the
mind-body-spirit framework.

- Green tea, for instance, is well-known for its anti-inflammatory properties due to the high concentration of catechins, which help reduce oxidative stress and promote cellular repair. This supports the body's natural healing process, especially in cases of chronic inflammation, which can be linked to emotional stress and unresolved trauma (Cao et al., 2017).
- Black tea, while containing caffeine, offers mental clarity and focus, supporting emotional balance by enhancing mood and providing an energy boost without the crash commonly associated with other stimulants.
- Herbal teas, such as chamomile and lavender, are rich in compounds that promote relaxation and reduce anxiety. These teas directly address

the emotional and nervous system imbalances often seen in individuals recovering from trauma (Zick et al., 2011).

- I have personally integrated these teas into my healing process as a form of microdosing, using them not just as a beverage but as a gentle, supportive supplement to restore balance. Consuming a variety of teas throughout the day allowed me to address both physical ailments, such as inflammation and digestive issues, and emotional struggles like anxiety and stress.
- The act of sipping tea itself became a grounding ritual—an opportunity to reconnect with my body and quiet my mind.
- By supplementing my routine with these teas, I was able to address both my physical and emotional well-being, providing consistent, small doses of healing throughout

the day, reinforcing my commitment to long-term recovery. In this way, teas not only supported my body's physical healing but also contributed to my emotional resilience, creating a layered, holistic approach to wellness (Sarris et al., 2013.)

15. REDUCE SUGAR (and artificial sweeteners) - A diet high in sugar has been linked to cognitive impairments and emotional issues such as anxiety and depression and leads to changes in brain function which alter emotional states and subsequent behaviors.
    - When sugar enters the body it gets broken down into glucose and fructose. GLUCOSE: is used immediately for energy production or stored for later. Insulin is released so the body can use the glucose. However, excessive glucose can't be broken down and used immediately because of insulin's interference, so it gets converted

into triglycerides. Some triglycerides get pushed out into circulation and may attach to vessel walls, while the remaining gets stored in the liver.....leading to a fatty liver.

- Artificial sweeteners are simply chemicals and will create a 'chemical response' in the body.
- Healthy sweetener options are: Honey, Maple Syrup, Monk Fruit and Agave.
  - Work to minimize the amount of sweetening agents you need to add to foods and beverages. As you reduce your sugar consumption you may notice the effects of sugar detox. This can be uncomfortable in the beginning, but the effects will recede over a short time.

16. SUGAR DETOX: Sugar works on the same receptors in the brain that opioids do, so it goes without saying that detoxing off of sugar can be "rough".

- Symptoms can include:

- Intense Sugar Cravings
- Headaches
- Muscle cramps and aches
- Nausea
- Irritability
- GI Issues
- Anxiety/Panic Attacks
- Joint Pain
- Sweats
- Depression

*This is not a complete list. The effects of sugar detox typically only last 3-7 days.

<u>Additional Modalities to Consider:</u>

<u>Essential Oils</u> - Find an aromatherapist to work with. Essential oils work on a physical and emotional level in the body.

The beauty of oils. You can use them for acute issues (colds, infections, yeast) or for more long-term issues. (immune support, releasing emotional issues, balancing. When using oils remember that they can be applied topically, diffused into the air or inhaled directly from the bottle or via an inhaler. For topical applications you can apply them *neat* (directly to the skin) or in a carrier oil. Preferably something natural and organic. (Coconut oil, Apricot oil, Jojoba, Olive, Grapeseed)

All oils have a vibrational frequency which makes them special and effective. When you add them to a synthetic oil or chemical it destroys that frequency and therefore can make them less effective. It is always wise to dilute the "hot" oils in a carrier oil until you know how you will react to them. ESPECIALLY if you are applying them to someone with sensitive skin, a child or the elderly.

<u>Using Essential Oils:</u>

- HOW: Always use your oils with PRAYER and INTENT. It will increase the natural frequency of the oils and enhance their effects.

- WHEN: Following the rule of 3 will have you using the oils #3 times a day for maintenance or chronic issues. If you are treating an acute issue or strong emotion, you may want to increase your applications to 7 times a day. 7 drops max and 3 drops minimum.

- WHERE: Always apply ON LOCATION. Or on the target area. As well as to the VitaFlex points on the hands and feet. Temple and base of the neck. Or utilize the 4 square breathing technique. (Works on the limbic system)

- WHO: Who can use essential oils? Anyone from infant to elderly. You can dilute the oils with a carrier oil such as coconut, jojoba, Almond or Olive oils. Do not mix them with synthetic oils/lotions/creams. This will cause the oils to lose their efficacy.

- WHY: God has given us something that can STAND ALONE or be used in conjunction with other medical treatments WITHOUT interacting. EO's can be used to boost the immune system, release blocked emotions, lift the mood, reset cells, heal, and flush toxins. Essential Oils can affect everything from your emotional state to your lifespan.

It is important to be CONSISTENT when using oils. It can take 3-6 months of daily use for a cellular shift to occur, but the changes that occur through oils are very natural and easy for the body.

<u>Crying Sessions</u> - Crying is a sign of normal and healthy emotional release. It can be seen as the beginning of processing the tough things in life. Research has found that crying activates the parasympathetic nervous system. This system helps your body return to a state of rest and digest.
Crying for long periods of time can release oxytocin. This chemical can help ease both physical and emotional pain.

<u>Exercise</u> - Some emotions are assisted in their release through activity. Here are some options that can facilitate the release of suppressed emotions.
- Yoga incorporates physical postures, breathing techniques, and meditation. Some yoga poses, like forward folds and twists, can help you let go of feelings that have been building up.
- Running or jogging: This type of exercise can help to release suppressed emotions

and tension. The pounding of feet on pavement or a treadmill can be therapeutic.
  - Resistance Training: Lifting weights can work as an effective way to release suppressed emotions.
  - High-intensity interval training (HIIT): HIIT is a type of exercise that alternates between high-intensity activity and rest. This is an effective way to release suppressed emotions and acute/chronic tension.
    - Boxing/Kickboxing classes can be useful in releasing certain types of emotion.

BIOFEEDBACK (EPR Stress Energetic Biofeedback)
EPR Stress Biofeedback is a method of measuring common physiological functions like skin temperature, heart rate, respiration, skin conductivity and muscle tension. This is done through reading over 26K body frequencies.

Biofeedback technicians and specialists are trained to use these signals to improve the wellness and wellbeing of their clients, and to support their lifestyle and health goals.

- May help determine the suppressed emotions and how they are impacting the body.

<u>Meditation</u> - Begin to meditate. It takes some effort. In the beginning you may only manage a few minutes but with time you will improve. If you struggle with what I call "monkey brain" start with 1-2 minutes and work up. Aim for a minimum of 15-30 minutes daily and increase as you become comfortable.

- <u>BioField Session</u> - Just like your circulatory and lymphatic systems need to flow, it is important that your energy is flowing as well. One way to do this is with BioField Sessions. This can be performed by a practitioner or you can do it yourself.
  - *See the instructions below*
- <u>Inner Child Meditation</u> - This is where you can do alot of SELF WORK.
  - Determining limiting self beliefs
  - Healing past hurts, trauma and misperceptions.
  - *See the instructions below*

<u>Massage</u> - Helps to increase serotonin and dopamine in the brain and decrease cortisol levels. This also stimulates and enhances the immune system.

- Deep tissue massage can often facilitate emotional release of negative emotions that have been stored in the body for years.
- Craniosacral massage techniques are also helpful with negative emotion release.

<u>Ozone therapy</u> - a holistic therapy that helps modulate the chemical balance in the body. It is a safe and natural way, without significant side effects, or potential for addiction. It does not interact with other medications.

Ozone affects the system as a whole by providing oxygenation of tissues, enhancing detox pathways, increasing circulation, enhancing the immune system, reducing pathogen load in the body, reducing oxidative stress, among many other ways.

- Ozone methods include: Skin application, insufflation (rectally or vaginally) mixing it with your blood and infusing it through an IV or by injection into tissue.
- Ozone also impacts the energy system of the body and can assist in helping

re-establish the mind/body disconnect and also in releasing suppressed emotions.

<u>FINALLY</u>:

- Don't push yourself
- Don't judge yourself
- Don't be hard on yourself
- Don't expect healing to take place all at once

This is a process. As you become more self-aware you will tailor the steps to your needs.

Meditations

Vitality Movement Method Meditation
(Self awareness Assessment)

In the beginning this will be easier if performed alone, in a quiet area, with no interruptions. This may feel very awkward or foreign at the start. When you have a mind/body disconnect it could very likely feel as if you are assessing someone ELSE's body, not your own. Keep going. Eventually you will begin to notice your body is 'waking up' inside.

The main focus of this practice is to get the energy in the body moving. Stagnant energy can be a factor in many issues and illnesses. Our bodies are flowing with energy. If our flow gets blocked it can cause a disruption or buildup. Energy flow is as important as circulation flow and lymphatic flow. Each plays a vital role in how the body works.

Once you get familiar with this approach and tuned in to your body and how it 'feels,' you will be able to do this meditation almost anywhere and it will become much easier.

- Pick a bible verse or affirmation phrase. *(Optional)*

- Find a quiet area. *(The best position to facilitate this is lying on your back in a frog position with the soles of your feet touching. However, you can modify this so it can be done in your car, your office, etc)*
- Begin by lying on your back in a frog position. The soles of your feet together, knees falling out to the sides.

  If you are unable to accommodate this position:

    1. *Try to lay with your knees bent so the soles of your feet on the ground.*
    2. *Lay with the soles of your feet against a wall, or piece of wooden furniture of possible*
- Close your eyes and slowly inhale deeply.
- Clear your mind. *(This may be difficult at first. You may find it difficult to slow the "monkey mind", stay with it. Over time you will find this is easier to manage.)*
- Place the fingertips of the right hand on the center of the crown of the head.
- Begin at your root center (placing your hand there or simply focusing on the area) Inhale for a count of 5-pause-exhale for a count of 8-pause. Repeat

this 3-5 times. *(You can repeat your verse or phrase at the end of each breath.)*

- Starting with the ROOT center. Place your left hand over the pubic bone. (Or anywhere along the root energy center line) Focus on inhaling fresh air into all of the endocrine organs associated with that center. Exhaling all negativity, suppressed emotions, etc. Each breath should be:

  > *Inhale for a count of 5 - pause - exhale for a count of 8 - pause, repeat x5 times for each energy center. If you are focusing on a verse or phrase you can repeat it at the end of each breath.*
  >
  > *If you have any known issues or ailments in this area, imagine the cells working to heal this problem. Oxygen is flowing in to heal and energize. The exhalation takes any debris or negative energy out and away. Remember - This is the breath of God flowing through your body. This meditation is best performed with prayer and supplication.*

- Move through each energy center, spending as much time on each area as you need to. Continue the breathwork, 5:8 breathing (*Inhale for a count*

*of 5 - pause - exhale for a count of 8 - pause) Focus
your prayer on the areas of need as you go.
(Physical and emotional)*

The energy centers are:

*Root center - at pubic bone
level*

*Sacral center - at the belly
button level*

*Solar center - at the stomach
level*

*Heart center - at the center
of the chest*

*Throat center - over the
thyroid*

*Pineal center - center of the
forehead*

Crown - top of the head

- When you reach the crown with your left hand, the next step is to place all fingertips on the center of the crown of the head. (The fingertips of the index, middle and ring fingers of BOTH hands will all be touching the crown.) Allow your breathing to return to normal. Allow your body to melt into whatever you are relaxing on. (bed, chair, floor)

- Focus on how your body feels.
  - Do you notice any areas where you have pain, tension, discomfort, heaviness, tightness, numbness, foreign feelings, darkness.
  - If so, focus your attention and breath into these areas. You can also apply a drop of an essential oil to this area.
  - *There is no WRONG WAY. This is YOUR practice. Do what feels right to you.*
- With your eyes still closed,
  - Allow yourself to return to your normal breathing.
  - Begin to wiggle your fingers and toes. Slowly move your arms and legs to begin to bring your body back to the present.
- Let your mind go quiet. You are relaxed. Let your body enjoy this state. *THIS is a healing state.*
- Open your eyes and remain in this relaxed state for as long as you can before resuming your day.

(This practice calms the nervous system, helping the body shift from fight-or-flight to rest-and-digest mode, which is essential for healing.)

Maintaining this state takes awareness, effort and consistency. When your body is in a relaxed state you have lower stress hormones in the body, you can digest your food better, your immune system improves, and your body can begin to recover and heal.

It is important that you work to maintain this healing state. If you are prone to anxiety, it is important that you work on your self awareness. When you find yourself in fight or flight (beginning to breathe more shallowly, tensing up, or any other symptoms of anxiety that you exhibit) take the time to focus on returning to a state of calm.

I have found during my own healing process I would select a bible verse or phrase that held truth for me in that phase of healing. I love *2 Corinthians 12:9, Jeremiah 29:11, Daniel 6:26 and 27*. I also like to implement phrases: *"Give me ears to listen and understand, and lips to respond effectively."* These would be focal points for my mind when I could feel myself escalating.

Sometimes it isn't possible to do a full assessment. You can modify the steps to help you return to calm.

Mindful Breathing Meditation

- Find a quiet space where you can sit comfortably.
- Close your eyes and take a deep breath.
- Begin to focus on your breathing: Inhale deeply for a count of four, hold for four, and exhale for six. Notice how your body feels as the breath flows in and out. If your mind wanders, gently bring your focus back to your breath.
- Close your eyes and take a deep breath.
  - Begin at your toes, noticing any sensations—warmth, tension, or relaxation.
  - Slowly move your attention upward through your legs, hips, back, and shoulders, pausing at each area.
  - If you notice tension or discomfort, breathe into that spot and imagine releasing it with each exhale.
- Move through your entire body with love and compassion.

- End by placing your hand over your heart, acknowledging your body with gratitude for all it does to support you.

Inner Child Meditation

(Assessment)

This meditation is best performed in an area where you feel safe to be vulnerable. *It's important that you have no interruptions. (other people, children, pets)*

As I said earlier, it may feel very awkward in the beginning. The beauty of this meditation is that you use the basic format, and you tailor it to your specific needs.

This form of self love also empowers you to be able to focus on mindfulness and being in the present... and no longer live in the past.

- Find a quiet place. Preferably where you will not be interrupted.
- Close your eyes and relax.
- Place the fingertips of the right hand on your crown and with the left hand you will start with the root energy center.

  Inhale for a count of 5 - pause - exhale for a count of 8 - pause, repeat x5 times for each energy center. Repeat this 4 times moving through each energy center until you reach the crown to bring the body to a calm centered feeling.

- Leaving the fingertips on the crown, place your left hand over the solar plexus.
- Imagine yourself when you were a child about four or five years old. See yourself as that child. Initially it may be difficult to do. Your mind will flutter and flicker. The goal is to BE CONSISTENT.
  - It may take you some time to learn to bring your mind to a state of calm before your younger self will emerge.
  - You may need to use a picture of yourself around this age to begin with.
- Once you are able to see yourself as a child, it is important to determine:
  - Are watching the events as if on a screen?
  - Are you present with your inner child, as if you were in the same room with them?
- Begin to investigate your feelings. Ask yourself:
  - *How do I feel about this child?*
  - *Do I love this child? Do I despise this child?*
  - *Do I find this child unworthy? Lonely? Unlovable? Terrified?*
  - *How would I describe this child?*

- ○ *WHO did this child have to turn to when they had serious fears, concerns or trouble? Who could they tell their deepest secrets to? (If you are unable to name anyone that you could confide the "deep stuff" to, this is not uncommon. That 'lack of security' often sets certain behaviors and defense mechanisms in place.)*
  - ○ *As you begin to establish what you BELIEVE about this child. Note that these are self limiting beliefs. (Self-limiting beliefs are perceptions that you have about yourself and about the way the world works. These assumptions are 'self-limiting' because in some way they're holding you back from achieving what you are capable of.)*
  - ○ *These beliefs are based on perception. NOT TRUTH.*
- Embrace this child, this younger you.
- *See them for who they are.* They are not the things that you have believed about them. Those perceptions and self limiting beliefs are only holding this child back from reaching their full potential.

- ○ *Hug this child.*
  - ○ *Talk to this child. Ask questions..... Ask what this child needs.*
  - ○ *Get to know this child. The more you understand this child, the more you will understand you. These are your deepest needs.*
- Acknowledge this child's fear, suffering, and pain so it feels both seen and heard.
- Thank this child for its vulnerability, its bravery, and its strength.
- Remember this child when you are practicing self-talk. Speak to yourself as if you were speaking to this child..... Tender, kind and with love.

- In the beginning this may be very difficult for you. To have an EMOTIONAL and vulnerable conversation with your 'SELF' may feel awkward or even SILLY.
  - ○ BE CONSISTENT. The more you practice it, the more you will reveal the unmet needs you have.
- The purpose of the "inner child meditation" is to help you work through your past issues, traumas, hurts, resentments, etc in a safe manner.

Consistency is KEY - The more you practice the process the more you will come to understand the effect of it. Our inner child is not always sitting there waiting for us. Especially if we are dealing with a lot of past hurts or abuse. It may even take a time or two (or 5) before we locate them.

To Clarify: *You are looking for yourself when you were about four or five years old. We usually find them in a place that was familiar and safe. It may be somewhere you are familiar with, or it may not.*

My Inner Child:

Many of the people I have spoken to that employ this meditation seem to always find their inner child in the same location. It may be in a treehouse, their childhood bedroom, at a grandparents home, at school, on the playground.

When I first began these meditations, I always found my five year old self in my kindergarten classroom. She was always sitting at the same table coloring.

(I can honestly say I never enjoyed school, in the whole 12 years that I went, it was not something I

looked forward to. Especially not my childhood kindergarten room. I liked my teacher, but that was such a terrifying time for me.

I didn't stay with babysitters as a child. I only interacted with my family. So for me to have to get on a bus alone, and go to school alone, was truly a terrifying action. I am still unclear as to why that is where she chooses to meet me. I'm sure she will divulge that information when the time is right.)

In the beginning it was as if I was watching her on a screen. Over time, it shifted and now, it is as if I am back in my kindergarten room WITH her. Initially she didn't speak. Sometimes she wouldn't even acknowledge that I was present. I really didn't know what to say in the beginning. So I just started trying to explain how her life had turned out.

Originally, I thought the goal was just to go back and tell her the story of her life and everything would turn out fine. So my initial meditations were basically me telling her the story of her life. How some of her perceptions had caused her much of the hurt/grief she experienced. It wasn't until I practiced the meditation several times and had gotten comfortable and familiar with the process that I realized there was much more involved.

When I first began the meditations, I thought that I felt sorry for that little girl. I pitied her. Truth be told, if asked, I would have told you that I didn't "love" her. I felt no affection towards her at all. I may have even said I "didn't like her". It was only after I had spent some time with her, in her world, coloring with her, talking to her.... I began to really look at her.... I saw her for who and what she was. A terrified, anxious and uncertain child. I began to feel this deep affection for her. I wanted to stop her from hurting. I wanted to lessen her pain. I wanted her to be happy. So I did less talking over my next couple of meditations, more coloring, and simply just watched her. I began to gain little insights through each meditation. I began to see her smile when I would talk about things. She really never spoke to me much, and she really didn't need to. Many times I just KNEW what her feelings and her needs were.

Each time I practiced the meditation something different would occur. Sometimes she would take my hand and we would walk out of my kindergarten classroom and into another scene of my life. Maybe it was something that happened when I was 14 years old. Maybe it was something that happened when I was 5 or 6. Many of these things I had forgotten about consciously, but they had all had some type of impact (good/bad) on my BE-ing.

I clearly recall one of my more intense meditations, a "break through" so to speak...
I asked her if she would show me her *deepest pain*. It was obvious that this was not something she wanted to do. She sat nervously for a little bit. And then she took me by the hand, and we walked out of the kindergarten classroom and into a funeral home. I recognized the location and knew this was going to be a difficult experience. She walked me to the side of the casket where my grandpa laid. Without saying anything, I knew her need. She had needed someone to explain the situation, to explain the pain and fear, to provide knowledge and understanding at a time when she couldn't comprehend what was happening around her. She needed someone to simply be there with her and hold her while she cried. And so I did.

She cried and cried and she finally began to process those emotions that had been buried so deep. *And so did I...*

We spent quite a bit of time there.I explained the situation to correct some of her misperceptions. I explained how her interpretation of the events have been so limited at her young age. I explained the facts of the events. I allowed her to stay there as long as she needed. As long as WE needed.

When the meditation ended, I could immediately feel a difference in my present body. I could feel a lightness that hadn't been there before. I could also feel the grief that I have spent so many years determined not to feel. The next couple of meditations found us back there. Each time we cried a little harder. At each meditation end, I found myself feeling a little lighter.

I don't want you to be discouraged, not all meditations are so serious. I have had several just sitting at the table coloring, and having a light conversation in which I did most of the talking. There have been a few times where we have found ourselves at the park, or the swimming pool, sometimes climbing trees. Occasionally we play with the toys that are there in the classroom. After all that's what kids love to do....PLAY!

I love to see her laugh. And I've come to realize even more, I LOVE HER. The exciting thing that you will come to realize, is the more you love this child, the more you
will love the person in the mirror. You will treat them kinder, you will be less judgmental with them, you will

find a new affection for them. As you love this child more, you will realize you are loving yourself.

Some meditations will only last 15 minutes. Others can last up to an hour. There is no end goal, or desired outcome from each meditation. What is *meant* to surface, *will* surface.

As I said, some of my meditations were simply just having fun. It's important to remember that you are allowing the thoughts, feelings, and events to surface without forcing them. To try and recall an upsetting event and picture yourself and your inner child there, *is not therapeutic*. It will not have the desired outcome. It may, in fact, cause more harm. If it is not time for you to address this, you will only be flooding your body with the hormones and emotions from that event as you "emotionally relive it". This is counterproductive.

This meditation practice is simply a means for you to do a deeper level of self work. A "self tool" that you can use to work on at your own pace. This is a means to reconnect with yourself. By loving this inner child can you begin to love yourself. Once you love yourself, then you can effectively love others.

There are MANY WAYS to Heal and Recover

You have to find the ways that resonate with YOU! Read books, listen to podcasts, talk to specialists.... It is important that you increase your knowledge and understanding. This will allow you to reach your goals in many different ways.

Healing is a process of gaining information and applying it. The more your knowledge base increases the better your overall understanding will be. You will begin to reach new levels of awareness and application.

Always remember.... This is YOUR LIFE! NO ONE has as much to lose as you do! NO ONE will be as committed to your recovery as YOU! Be your own advocate and don't settle.

When I began my journey, I had NO IDEA what I was doing. It was truly trial and error. Some modalities produced better outcomes than others. Some caused me to struggle with focus, however, in time I conquered my "monkey brain" issues and found these practices helped with my anger and aggression issues.

By no means am I HEALED. Like I stated earlier, healing is PROCESS not an "end result'. It is an ongoing journey. One that will become lighter and easier as you continue. It will become a 'way of life'.

I started my journey when I turned 43yrs. I can honestly say I am HEALTHIER now at 50 yrs than I was at 38 yrs. I have less pain, less GI issues, less brain fog. I have a stronger intuition, constitution and mindset. My self awareness is stronger and I find it easier to FEEL and process my emotions.

I still have a long way to go, but I am confident and excited to continue on my path. I am also CERTAIN that if I can do this, anyone can change their life!
The time is NOW!
What do you have to lose? Only your health, your vitality, and ultimately your LIFE. Those options were unacceptable to me, I am sure they are to YOU as well.

As I said before, I followed a bread crumb trail. My goal is to provide you with initial direction to get you started. To provide you with useful knowledge and deeper understanding as you navigate through your feelings and emotions. The remaining pages are for your notes. Hopefully this will help you get a jumpstart on your own journey, you are beginning a process that will change the rest of your life.

Love and Best Wishes on your journey....

-xoxo- Angel

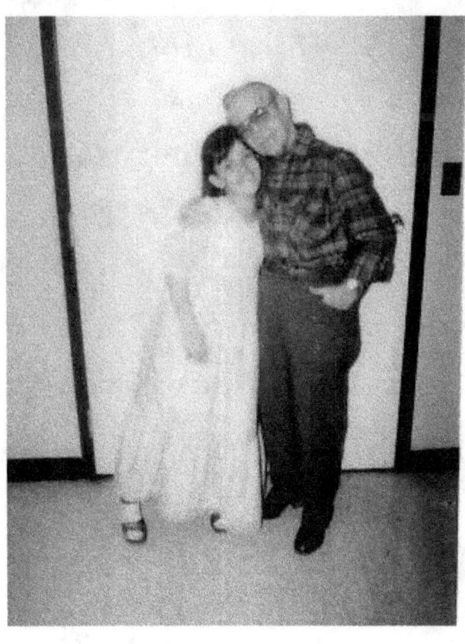

References:

van der Kolk, B. (2014). *The Body Keeps the Score: Brain, Mind, and Body in the Healing of Trauma.* Penguin Books.

Cohen, S., Janicki-Deverts, D., & Miller, G. E. (2012). "Psychological Stress and Disease." *JAMA Internal Medicine.*

Winston, D., & Maimes, S. (2007). Adaptogens: Herbs for Strength, Stamina, and Stress Relief. Healing Arts Press.

Winston, D., & Maimes, S. (2007). Adaptogens: Herbs for Strength, Stamina, and Stress Relief. Healing Arts Press.

Gerin, W., Davidson, K. W., et al. (2012). "The Role of Stress-Induced Emotions in Heart Disease." Nature Reviews Cardiology.